数据管理能力框架

Data Management Competency Framework

编　写　世界卫生组织
编　译　国家卫生健康委统计信息中心

中国协和医科大学出版社
北　京

著作权合同登记　图字：01-2024-2672号

世界卫生组织于2023年发布，标题为《数据管理能力框架》

◎世界卫生组织，2023年

世界卫生组织总干事已将中文版的翻译权授予中国国家卫生健康委员会统计信息中心，由该中心全权负责翻译工作。

图书在版编目（CIP）数据

数据管理能力框架 / 世界卫生组织编；国家卫生健康委统计信息中心编译. —北京：中国协和医科大学出版社，2024.5

书名原文：Data Management Competency Framework

ISBN 978-7-5679-1531-2

Ⅰ.①数…　Ⅱ.①世…　②国…　Ⅲ.①医药卫生管理－信息管理　Ⅳ.①R19

中国国家版本馆CIP数据核字（2024）第083365号

编　　写	世界卫生组织
编　　译	国家卫生健康委统计信息中心
策　　划	杨　帆
责任编辑	高淑英
封面设计	邱晓俐
责任校对	张　麓
责任印制	黄艳霞
出版发行	中国协和医科大学出版社
	（北京市东城区东单三条9号　邮编100730　电话010-65260431）
网　　址	www.pumcp.com
印　　刷	北京捷迅佳彩印刷有限公司
开　　本	787mm×1092mm　　1/16
印　　张	11.25
字　　数	160千字
版　　次	2024年5月第1版
印　　次	2024年5月第1次印刷
定　　价	89.00元

译者名单

主 译

吴士勇　国家卫生健康委统计信息中心

译 者（按姓氏笔画排序）

吴士勇　国家卫生健康委统计信息中心

邱　月　清华大学医院管理研究院

何　平　北京大学中国卫生发展研究中心

张耀光　国家卫生健康委统计信息中心

陈俐锦　国家卫生健康委统计信息中心

周忠良　西安交通大学公共政策与管理学院

赵亚楠　北京大学中国卫生发展研究中心

胡广宇　中国医学科学院医学信息研究所

洪　颖　北京大学第一医院

潘　杰　四川大学华西公共卫生学院 / 华西第四医院

Data management competency framework

© World Health Organization 2023

ISBN 978 9 29062 009 9

推荐引用. Data management competency framework. Manila. World Health Organization Regional Office for the Western Pacific. 2023. Licence：CC BY-NC-SA 3.0 IGO..

出版编目（CIP）数据 . 1. Data management. 2. Data management system. 3. Health information management. I. World Health Organization Regional Office for the Western Pacific.（NLM Classification：W26.55.I3） third-party-owned component in the work rests solely with the user.

General disclaimers. The designations employed and the presentation of the material in this publication do not imply the expression of any opinion whatsoever on the part of WHO concerning the legal status of any country, territory, city or area or of its authorities, or concerning the delimitation of its frontiers or boundaries. Dotted and dashed lines on maps represent approximate border lines for which there may not yet be full agreement.

The mention of specific companies or of certain manufacturers' products does not imply that they are endorsed or recommended by WHO in preference to others of a similar nature that are not mentioned. Errors and omissions excepted, the names of proprietary products are distinguished by initial capital letters.

All reasonable precautions have been taken by WHO to verify the information contained in this publication. However, the published material is being distributed without warranty of any kind, either expressed or implied. The responsibility for the interpretation and use of the material lies with the reader. In no event shall WHO be liable for damages arising from its use.

Photo credits: © WHO/Yoshi Shimizu, pp. iv, 3, 33, 45; © WHO/Mengjuan Duan, p. vii; © WHO/Muhd Ikmal Photography pp. 21, 39, 47;

© WHO/Jason Chute, p. 25; © WHO/Until Chan pp. 34, 37; © WHO/Tytaart p. 49; © WHO/Silifaiga Luuni, p. 52.

第三方材料。如果您希望重复使用本作品中属于第三方的材料，如表格、图形或图像，您有责任确定重复使用是否需要许可，并获得版权持有人的许可。作品中任何第三方拥有的组件受到侵犯而导致索赔的风险完全由用户承担。

一般免责声明。本出版物中使用的名称和材料的介绍并不意味着世界卫生组织对任何国家、领土、城市或地区或其当局的法律地位，或对其边界或边界的划定发表任何意见。地图上的点划线表示可能尚未完全达成一致的边界线。

提及特定公司或某些制造商的产品并不意味着世界卫生组织认可或推荐这些公司或制造商的产品。除错误和遗漏外，专有产品的名称以首字母大写区分。

世界卫生组织已采取一切合理的预防措施，以核实本出版物所包含的信息。出版的内容在没有任何明示或暗示保证的情况下进行出版。解读和使用材料的责任在于读者。在任何情况下，世界卫生组织均不对其使用造成的损害承担责任。

图片来源：© WHO/Yoshi Shimizu，pp. iv，3，33，45；© WHO/Mengjuan Duan，p. vii；© WHO/Muhd Ikmal Photography pp. 21，39，47；© WHO/Jason Chute，p. 25；© WHO/Until Chan pp. 34，37；© WHO/Tytaart p. 49；© WHO/Silifaiga Luuni，p. 52.

译者前言

    数据已经成为一种基本生产要素和核心战略资源，科学、系统、及时的数据应用是国家治理体系和治理能力现代化的重要支撑。卫生健康数据具有数据量大、结构复杂、类型众多、价值大、技术要求高等特点，其收集、分析和应用更是政策制定和研究者高度关注的问题。

    中国已经构建了覆盖各级各类医疗卫生机构的数据收集体系，积累了覆盖全人群、全生命周期的医疗健康数据。通过对上述数据的分析和利用，有效支撑了卫生健康相关的管理决策、行业监管以及科学研究，为健康中国建设和积极应对人口老龄化国家战略提供了信息支持。

    中国建立了包括卫生健康行政部门、医疗卫生机构以及科研院校等机构的专职、兼职统计和信息专业人员队伍。如何对卫生统计、信息专业人才开展系统的能力评估，并根据评估的结果有针对性地开展培训、培养，促进卫生健康统计、信息队伍建设的可持续、高质量发展，提高数据应用和管理能力，更好地发挥数据价值，成为卫生健康工作的重要议题。

    世界卫生组织西太区制定了《数据管理能力框架》，从知识维度、技能维度及态度维度，构建了涵盖数据生成、清理、分析和应用的全流程的能力框架，并将知识和技能维度分为初级学习者、新手从业者、独立从业者和高级从业者，对于不同层级的专业人员有针对性地提出了其应该具备的知识和技能。该框架对于加强统计和信息化专业人员的能力建设具有较好的参考价值。

    国家卫生健康委统计信息中心与世界卫生组织共同成立了世界卫生组织卫生信息与信息学合作中心，旨在加强数据治理、应用以及数字健康的国际交流、合作，促进相关领域的知识共享。为介绍国际数据管理与应用的理念和方法，经过世界卫生组织的授权，我们引进并组织翻译了《数据管理能力框架》，为进一步推进中国卫生健康数据的管理和应用提供借鉴。

《数据管理能力框架》可以作为各级卫生健康统计信息机构以及医疗卫生机构统计、信息、数据分析等部门以及科研院所、技术企业评价和提升数据管理能力的参考资料，也可以在机构的设置、人员招聘、培养培训、选拔晋升等方面参考使用。

为便于读者对照阅读、使用，我们采用了原文与译文双语对应的方式进行排版。翻译难免存在疏漏以及不足，敬请读者批评指正。

国家卫生健康委统计信息中心

2023年11月

Foreword

The needs of data-driven global and national strategies call for a rethinking of the way data are managed and how we use data with purpose. New technologies have accelerated growth in data types, volumes and complexity. Complicated and emerging health challenges that impact both social and economic environments simultaneously require maximizing the use of data for strategic dialogue and decision-making.

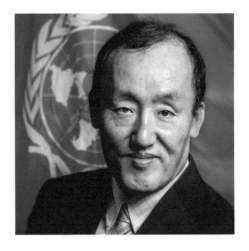

The health information management profession has been making a vital contribution to supporting health care and health-care delivery. With new demands comes the requirement for the health information workforce (HIW) to stay abreast of these changes in terms of what they mean for their roles. However, there remains a significant divergence across the globe in the levels of HIW education, training and development environments and the levels of professionalization, resulting in wide variations and differences in the levels of work readiness among graduates preparing to enter the workforce.

The World Health Organization (WHO) Regional Office for the Western Pacific, with support from WHO country offices and headquarters and in collaboration with partner organizations, is pleased to present the *Data Management Competency Framework*, a tool that provides a clear definition of each component of the data life cycle as well as the required skills and knowledge for different HIW levels, thus providing the capability to identify current competency gaps, measure competency development and identify future competency needs to support Member States in promoting sustainable and integrated capacity-building for both the

序

数据驱动的全球和国家战略，需要重新审视数据管理方式以及数据使用的目的。新技术加速并丰富了数据类型、数量和复杂性。复杂而新兴的健康挑战能够同时影响社会和经济环境，面对这种复杂的局面，需要最大化利用数据开展战略对话和决策制定。

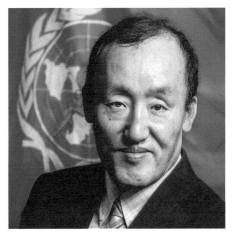

卫生信息管理领域一直在为支持医疗卫生服务体系和服务提供做出重要贡献。随着新的需求出现，卫生信息专业人员需要紧跟这些变化，了解这些变化有助于发挥其作用。然而，在全球范围内，卫生信息专业人员在受教育水平、培训程度、发展环境和专业化程度方面存在显著差异，导致进入这一行业的专业人员的知识储备和工作能力存在较大差距。

世界卫生组织（WHO）西太平洋区域办事处在各国代表处和总部的支持下，与伙伴组织紧密合作，很高兴出版《数据管理能力框架》。本书清晰定义了数据生命周期的各个环节、不同层次卫生信息专业人员所需的技能和知识，从而识别当前能力差距、衡量能力发展和预测未来能力需要，以支持成员国在短期和长期内推动可持续的、综合的能力建设。

short and longer terms.

The Framework is a comprehensive, practical guide that Member States can adapt to suit their own circumstances and their own vision and goals. Its publication is very timely, coinciding with the requirement to align the changing environment with the need for utilization of multiple data resources. This is a period, especially due to the coronavirus disease (COVID-19) pandemic, when all health systems face stringent health challenges, greater demands for efficiencies and higher expectations of health information.

This Framework expertly demonstrates how to take action now to achieve strategic, sustainable and integrated capacity-building for all HIW levels and types of health institutions in a tailored way. While it brings decision-makers, managers, implementors and front-line health workers at national and subnational levels much closer together, the Framework also encourages and provides the opportunity for active multi-stakeholder collaboration, including both horizontal approaches between different departments and their human resource departments, as well as vertical approaches across national, provincial, district and health-centre levels.

Dr Kidong Park, M.D., Ph.D.
Director
Data, Strategy and Innovation (DSI)
WHO Regional Office for the Western Pacific

这个框架是一份全面的、实用性的指南，成员国可以根据自己的情况、愿景和目标进行调整和应用。它的发布非常及时，能够与需要利用多种数据资源且时刻处在变化之中的环境要求相吻合。特别是在新型冠状病毒感染（COVID-19）大流行的背景下，所有卫生体系都面临更严峻的健康挑战、更高的效率要求和卫生健康信息的更高期望。

这个框架专业地展示了如何立即采取行动，以量身定制的方式为所有不同层级的卫生信息专业人员和不同类型的机构实现战略性、可持续性和综合性的能力建设。它能够使得国家和地方各级的决策者、管理者、执行者和一线卫生专业人员更加紧密地协作，同时能够鼓励提供积极的、多利益相关者的合作机会，包括不同机构、部门之间的水平协作，以及国家级、省级、地区级和基层医疗卫生机构之间的垂直协作。

Dr Kidong Park，M.D.，Ph.D.
司长
数据、战略与创新司（DSI）
世界卫生组织（WHO）西太平洋区域办事处

Acknowledgements

The *Data Management Competency Framework* was developed under the guidance of Dr Kidong Park, Director of the Data, Strategy and Innovation (DSI) Group at the World Health Organization (WHO) Regional Office for the Western Pacific, and Dr Gao Jun, Team Coordinator, Health Information and Intelligence unit (HII) of DSI.

The core writing group members consisted of Mengjuan Duan, Eugene O'Curry and Robert Arciaga from HII.

Technical inputs at the conceptualization stage were provided by Brian Riley, Vladimir Choi, Roberta Pastore, Priya Mannava, Linh-Vi Le, Fukushi Morishita and Elena Dolmat from the WHO Regional Office for the Western Pacific.

Further technical inputs were provided at the drafting stage by Ana Mendez-Lopez, Tracy Yuen, Linh-Vi Le, Fukushi Morishita and Josaia Tiko from the WHO Regional Office for the Western Pacific; Roland Dilipkumar Hensman, Phatsaline Vongsaly, Carl Massonneau, Hiroko Henker, Daisuke Asai, Khamphao Keonantatilard and Vilath Seevisay from the WHO country office in the Lao People's Democratic Republic; and Hong Anh Chu, Doris Ma Fat, Nenad Kostanjsek, Nelly Biondi, Luhua Zhao, Bochen Cao and Derrick Muneene from WHO headquarters.

Contributions to the Papua New Guinea case story were provided by Sevil Huseynova, Priya Mannava, Anna Maalsen and Getinet Adenager from the WHO country office in Papua New Guinea and Manah Dindi from the National Department of Health, Papua New Guinea.

The draft *Data Management Competency Framework* was reviewed by the following external technical experts: Vicki Bennett, Filippa Pretty, Nicola Richards, Georgia Savvopoulos, Ashna Kumar, Kate Spyby, Brooke Macpherson, Breanna Harnetty, Miriam Lum On and Ashleigh Bennett from the Australia Institute of Health and Welfare; Willy Chan from the New South Wales Local Health

致　谢

《数据管理能力框架》是在世界卫生组织（WHO）西太平洋区域数据、战略与创新司（DSI）司长 Kidong Park 博士和卫生信息与情报部（HII）协调员 Gao Jun 博士的指导下编著的。

核心编写团队成员包括来自 HII 的 Mengjuan Duan、Eugene O'Curry 和 Robert Arciaga。

世界卫生组织西太平洋区域办事处的 Brian Riley、Vladimir Choi、Roberta Pastore、Priya Mannava、Linh-Vi Le、Fukushi Morishita 和 Elena Dolmat 在概念框架阶段提供技术支持。

世界卫生组织西太平洋区域办事处 Ana Mendez-Lopez, Tracy Yuen, Linh-Vi Le，Fukushi Morishita 和 Josaia Tiko，世界卫生组织驻老挝人民民主共和国办事处 Roland Dilipkumar Hensman, Phatsaline Vongsaly, Carl Massonneau, Hiroko Henker, Daisuke Asai, Khamphao Keonantatilard 和 Vilath Seevisay。世界卫生组织总部 Hong Anh Chu, Doris Ma Fat, Nenad Kostanjsek, Nelly Biondi, Luhua Zhao, Bochen Cao 和 Derrick Muneene 在起草框架阶段提供了进一步的技术支持。

世界卫生组织巴布亚新几内亚办事处 Sevil Huseynova, Priya Mannava, Anna Maalsen 和 Getinet Adenager 以及该国卫生部的 Manah Dindi 提供了案例。

《数据管理能力框架》的稿件还得到了以下外部技术专家的审查：澳大利亚卫生福利研究所的 Vicki Bennett、Filippa Pretty、Nicola Richards、Georgia Savvopoulos、Ashna Kumar、Kate Spyby、Brooke Macpherson、Breanna Harnetty、Miriam Lum On 和 Ashleigh Bennett，来自新南威尔士州地方卫生局的 Willy Chan，来自圣文森特健康澳大利亚的 Cameron Barnes，来自格

District; Cameron Barnes from St Vincent's Health Australia; Sheree Lloyd from the Griffith University and University of Tasmania; and Louise Edmonds from Calvary.

里菲斯大学和塔斯马尼亚大学的Sheree Lloyd以及来自加尔文医院的Louise Edmonds。

Abbreviations

ANOVA	analysis of variance（statistical technique）
COVID-19	coronavirus disease
CAPI	computer-assisted personal interview
DHIS2	District Health Information System 2
DBMS	database management system
DSI	Data，Strategy and Innovation（Group）
ELT	extract，load and transform
ETL	extract，transform and load
FHIR	Fast Healthcare Interoperability Resources
GIS	geographic information system
HIW	health information workforce
HIS	health information system
HR	human resource
INLA	integrated nested Laplace approximation
ISO	International Organization for Standardization
KTA	Knowledge to Action
MDR-TB	multidrug-resistant tuberculosis
M&E	monitoring and evaluation
R	（programme scripting language）
RHIS	routine health information system
SMART	specific，measurable，achievable，relevant，time-bound
SOP	standard operating procedure

缩　写

ANOVA	方差分析（统计技术）
COVID-19	新型冠状病毒感染
CAPI	计算机辅助访谈
DHIS2	地区卫生信息系统2
DBMS	数据库管理系统
DSI	数据、战略与创新（小组）
ELT	提取、加载、转换
ETL	提取、转换、加载
FHIR	快速医疗互操作性资源
GIS	地理信息系统
HIW	卫生信息专业人员
HIS	卫生信息系统
HR	人力资源
INLA	集成嵌套拉普拉斯近似法
ISO	国际标准化组织
KTA	知识转化行为
MDR-TB	耐多药肺结核
M&E	监测和评估
R	（统计编程脚本语言）
RHIS	常规卫生信息系统
SMART	具体的、可测量的、可实现的、相关的、时限性的
SOP	标准操作规程

SAS	statistical analysis software
SDGs	Sustainable Development Goals
SPSS	Statistical Package for the Social Sciences
SQL	structured query language
WHO	World Health Organization

SAS	统计分析软件
SDGs	可持续发展目标
SPSS	社会科学统计软件包
SQL	结构化查询语言
WHO	世界卫生组织

Executive Summary

The effective use of data in the management and delivery of public health services has long been understood as critical by public health professionals. Over recent decades, countries have made significant investments in the improvement of data generation and quality, but mostly from the perspective of data generation rather than that of data users. New technologies have accelerated growth in data types, volumes and complexity. Emerging and complicated health challenges that impact both social and economic environments simultaneously require maximizing the use of data for strategic dialogue and decision-making.

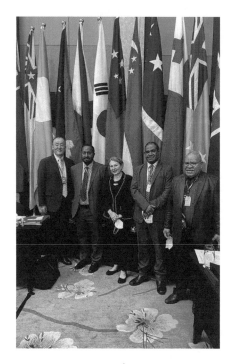

With new demands comes the requirement for the health information workforce (HIW) to stay abreast of these changes in terms of what they mean for their roles. Developing the range of human competencies necessary to understand and interpret the ever-changing risks to and complexities of public health through the effective use of data management skills remains an ongoing challenge in many countries. There remains a significant divergence across the globe in the levels of HIW education, training and development environments and the levels of employee professionalization, resulting in wide variations and differences in the levels of work readiness among graduates preparing to enter the workforce. These changing needs and expectations call for a rethinking of the way data are managed and how we use data with purpose.

长期以来，公共卫生专业人员一直认为，在公共卫生服务的管理和提供中，有效利用数据是至关重要的。在过去的几十年里，各国在数据生成和质量改进方面进行了大量投资，但主要是从数据生成的角度，而不是基于数据使用者的角度。新技术的发展加速并丰富了数据类型、数量和复杂性。新兴而复杂的健康挑战同时影响社会和经济环境，需要最大限度地利用数据进行战略对话和决策。

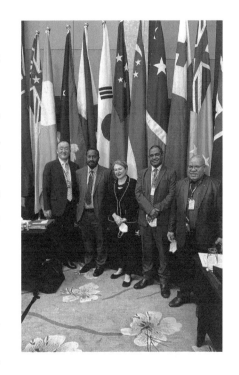

随着新的需求不断增长，卫生信息专业人员（HIW）需要及时了解这些变化对他们意味着什么。通过有效使用数据管理技能，发展人们理解和解释公共卫生不断变化的风险和复杂性所需的各种能力，这在许多国家仍然是一项持续的挑战。在全球范围内，卫生信息专业人员在受教育水平、培训程度、发展环境和专业化程度方面存在显著差异，导致进入这一行业的专业人员知识储备和工作能力存在较大差距。

To address this challenge, the Data, Strategy and Innovation (DSI) Data Group was set up to lead office-wide collaboration on key health information priorities with "data focal points" across all divisions of the World Health Organization (WHO) Regional Office for the Western Pacific. In collaboration with a team of WHO colleagues from headquarters and country offices, external partners and experts, the Data Group has designed and developed the *Data Management Competency Framework* as a practical tool to provide both a structure and methodology to enable HIW employees (who have cause and need to engage with health data), their line managers and human resource (HR) managers to define the competencies required for the identified data management roles within their organizations. The value and benefits deriving from the use of the Framework are numerous and varied. They range from identifying individual, unit, department and divisional competency gaps and training needs at an operational level, to informing and guiding employee recruitment and selection, training and development, and team formation at an organizational level.

The Framework is designed around the four core stages of the data management cycle: data generation, processing, analysis and usage. Within the Framework, these stages are classified as competency areas, and within these four competency areas, a further 17 competency domains have been identified. These domains are effectively sets of sub-competencies within the wider competency areas. The Framework provides users with detailed domain definitions and specific descriptors of the technical knowledge and skill sets covered within each domain. The Framework further provides and describes four proficiency levels, i.e. levels of competence within each domain, and describes the technical knowledge and skills that determine the achievement of each proficiency level. This is rounded out by attitudinal domains that describes behaviours and mindsets that are essential for long-term sustainable capacity-building.

The Framework provides in-country management, for the first time, with a detailed, comprehensive, integrated and coherent tool to define and assess current and future competency needs for their HIW. The objective in producing and introducing this Framework is to make it the go-to competency mapping and development tool for health information employees, their line managers and HR managers across the WHO Western Pacific Region. Using the Framework comprehensively and consistently will yield a host of benefits for the HIW.

As with all organizational change initiatives, the key to success is effective implementation. Local ownership of and responsibility for implementation are critical. Country management must embrace the concept and put in place the necessary oversight and implementation structures to ensure successful adoption. This document describes a seven-step process to guide those entrusted with responsibility for implementation.

为应对这一挑战，成立了数据、战略和创新（DSI）数据团队，承担了协调世界卫生组织西太平洋区域办事处在关键卫生信息优先领域（"数据集中点"）的跨部门协作工作。DSI数据团队与世界卫生组织总部和国家办事处的同事、外部合作伙伴和专家合作设计和开发了《数据管理能力框架》。作为一个实用工具，它为信息专业人员（需要与健康数据打交道的人员）、他们的部门负责人和人力资源负责人提供了一种结构和方法，以定义其组织内所需的数据管理角色的能力要求。使用该框架能够带来大量且多维度的价值，在执行层面可以识别个人、单位和部门的能力差距和培训需求，在组织层面可以指导员工招聘、选拔、培训和发展以及团队的组建。

该框架围绕数据管理流程的四个核心阶段设计，分别为数据生成、处理、分析和应用。该框架将这些阶段分为四个能力领域，进而确定了17个能力维度。这些能力维度是由更广泛的子能力构成的。此外，该框架还提供给使用者清晰的针对各个维度的定义，同时也详细描述了每个维度内技术性的知识和技能。此外，该框架还为每个维度提供4个不同的熟练水平，并描述了实现每个熟练水平所需要的技术知识和技能。最后，包括了态度维度的问题，描述了对于长期可持续的能力建设至关重要的行为和思维方式。

该框架首次提供了一个内部管理工具，能够详细、全面、综合和一致地用于定义和评估卫生信息专业人员（HIW）的现在和未来的能力需求。制定并引入此框架的目标是使其成为世界卫生组织西太平洋区域内卫生信息专业人员、部门负责人和人力资源负责人的能力指南和发展的首选工具。全面且一致使用该框架，将为卫生信息专业人员带来一系列益处。

与所有组织变革项目一样，成功的关键在于有效的实施。当地的权力和责任对于实施至关重要。各国层面的管理层需要接受并认同这一概念，并建立必要的监督和实施框架，以确保成功。本书阐述了包含七个步骤的过程，以指导负责实施的人员。

目录 Contents

目录 Contents

1. Introduction

1. 前言

■ Background

Accurate, reliable and timely data are critical for driving global and national health strategies and for ensuring the advancement of national health goals in Member States of the World Health Organization (WHO) Western Pacific Region, while simultaneously meeting internationally agreed commitments such as the health-related Sustainable Development Goals (SDGs). Over recent decades, countries have made significant investments in the improvement of their health information systems (HIS) to respond to the ever-increasing demands for new and better data. Due to the coronavirus disease (COVID-19) pandemic, decision-makers and broader populations have recognized the importance of resilient and robust HIS, with a trend of increased investments over the past two years (1). Multiple digital tools and platforms have been developed or embedded into current systems in Member States (2).

A common challenge, however, is that health information workforces (HIWs) do not have the robust capacities to participate in data generation, processing, analysis and usage in a reliable, consistent and timely manner, which minimizes the impact of investments made in HIS development.

The development of HIW capacity is lagging behind the continuous improvement of HIS, especially since the COVID-19 pandemic. There are large variances in the roles, responsibilities and competencies across the HIW, both within and between countries (3). Capacity-building initiatives and activities normally follow traditional, fragmented and ad hoc approaches (Fig. 1), which regularly result in suboptimal and non-sustainable investment returns.

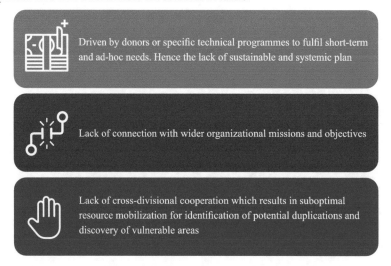

Driven by donors or specific technical programmes to fulfil short-term and ad-hoc needs. Hence the lack of sustainable and systemic plan

Lack of connection with wider organizational missions and objectives

Lack of cross-divisional cooperation which results in suboptimal resource mobilization for identification of potential duplications and discovery of vulnerable areas

Fig. 1　Common challenges for traditional capacity-building

■背景

　　准确、可靠和及时的数据对于推动全球和国家卫生战略以及确保世界卫生组织西太平洋地区成员国推进国家卫生目标，同时履行与卫生相关的可持续发展目标等国际商定承诺至关重要。近几十年来，各国在改进卫生信息系统（HIS）方面进行了大量投资，以满足对新数据和更好数据日益增长的需求。由于新型冠状病毒感染的流行，决策者和更多的人已经认识到有韧性的和强健的卫生信息系统的重要性，在过去两年中对卫生信息系统投资呈增加趋势[1]。成员国开发了多种数字工具和平台，或将其嵌入到现有系统中[2]。

　　然而，一个共同的挑战是，卫生信息人力资源（HIW）不具备可靠、一致和及时地参与数据生成、处理、分析和应用的强大能力，这就最大限度地降低了对卫生信息系统发展所做投资的影响。

　　特别是自新型冠状病毒感染疫情大流行以来，卫生信息人力资源能力的发展落后于卫生信息系统的不断改进。无论是在同一国家内部还是在不同国家之间，卫生信息人力资源的作用、职责和能力都存在很大差异[3]。能力建设倡议和活动通常采用传统、分散和临时的方法（图1），结果往往是投资回报不理想且不可持续。

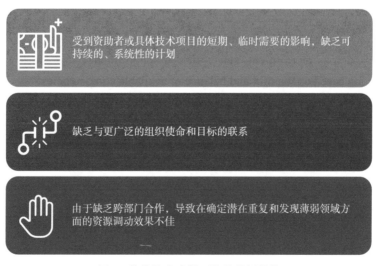

图1　传统能力建设面临的共同挑战

As a first step in addressing these systemic weaknesses, the WHO Regional Office for the Western Pacific created a cross-functional, multidisciplinary Data Group to devise and implement an overarching strategic response to this problem. Within this group of specialists, a Capacity-Building Working Group was formed to lead the design and development of a systematic and integrated approach to strengthening the HIW capacity of Member States at different levels and types of health institutions. The outcome of these efforts, in collaboration with a mixed team of WHO colleagues from headquarters and country offices, external partners and experts, is this *Data Management Competency Framework*, which is described in more detail on the following pages.

■ Objective

The Framework is an essential tool for health information management teams in Member States to identify capacity gaps and plan and drive the competency development of their HIW across different levels of their health institutions and organizations. More specifically, it is a reference tool for activities that can:

· measure the skill and knowledge gaps of individuals or homogeneous role types within the HIW at each step of the data life cycle (Fig. 2);

· identify and specify the required skills and knowledge within the workforce to match current roles and responsibilities;

· identify and map the priority areas for both short and long-term training and development planning at the individual, unit, department and division level within the HIW in the organization; and

· inform, guide and support strategic human resources (HR) management activities such as recruitment, selection and appointments, team formation and composition based on the mix and balance of available competencies.

■ Target audiences

The principal target audiences for the Framework are the line and HR management teams from Member States to enable them to create data management competency profiles (required and actual) for their health information employees. Such roles would typically include but are not limited to:

· decision-makers, managers, implementors and front-line health workers who develop, manage and use HIS, such as health and clinical information professionals and officers;

作为解决这些系统性缺陷的第一步，世界卫生组织西太平洋区域办事处成立了一个跨职能、多学科数据小组，以制定和实施解决这一问题的总体战略对策。在这个专家小组内，成立了一个能力建设工作组，领导设计和制定系统的综合方法，以加强成员国在不同级别和类型卫生机构的卫生信息专业人员的工作能力。通过与世界卫生组织总部和国家办事处的同事、外部合作伙伴和专家组成的多元化团队合作，这些努力的成果就是本数据管理能力框架，下文将对其进行更详细的介绍。

■ 目标

该框架是成员国卫生信息管理团队确定能力差距、制定规划和推动卫生信息专业人员能力发展的重要工具。具体来说，它是开展以下活动的参考工具：

· 在数据生命周期的每一个步骤中，衡量卫生信息专业人员个人及同质角色类型的技能和知识差距（图2）。

· 明确卫生信息专业人员所需的技能和知识，以匹配当前的角色和职责。

· 确定组织内个人、单位、部门和分部的短期和长期培训与发展规划的优先领域。

· 告知、指导和支持战略性人力资源管理活动，如基于综合的、平衡的能力进行招聘、遴选、任命和团队组建。

■ 目标受众

该框架的主要目标受众是成员国的卫生信息业务管理人员和人力资源管理人员，使其能够为卫生信息专业人员建立数据管理能力档案（内容含实际能力和必需能力）。这些角色通常包括但不限于：

· 开发、管理和使用卫生信息系统的决策者、管理者、执行者和一线卫生专业人员，如卫生和临床信息专业人员和管理人员。

·decision-makers, managers, implementors and front-line health workers who input data and extract information for routine work, such as specific disease-control managers, records managers, surveillance and monitoring officers, and data analysts; and

·adoption/implementation leaders and influencers, such as national and subnational health system decision-makers, front-line functional line managers, HR managers and training managers.

·Software designers and information technology specialists are not included.

■ Framework structure and components

The Framework (illustrated in Fig. 2) is designed around four competency areas or "pillars" that are based on the four stages of the data management cycle: data generation, processing, analysis and usage. Within each competency area are competency domains (17 domains in total), which are distinct and essential sub-competencies. Within each competency domain, there are three competency dimensions (subject knowledge, practical skills and personal attitude), which, when combined, determine the overall level of competence of an individual employee.

Knowledge and skills are further categorized into four proficiency levels (ranging from learner-beginner to master practitioner), which describe the varying degrees of proficiency achievable for each domain. Attitudes are further categorized into attitudinal domains which collectively describe behaviours and mindsets which create an environment of excellence and respect leading to long-term sustainable capacity-building. Details can be found in the following chapter.

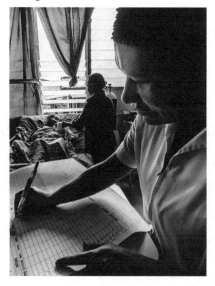

·日常工作需要输入数据和提取信息的决策者、管理者、执行者和一线卫生专业人员，如具体的疾病控制管理人员、数据记录管理人员、监测人员和数据分析师。

·实施工作的领导者和有影响力的人，如国家级和次国家级卫生体系的决策者、一线职能部门的管理人员、人力资源负责人和培训管理者。

·软件设计师和信息技术专家不包括在内。

■ 框架结构与组成

该框架（图2）围绕四个能力领域或"支柱"设计，以数据管理周期的四个阶段为基础：数据生成、处理、分析和使用。每个能力领域内都有能力维度（共17个维度），这是不同的基本子能力。在每个能力领域中，有三个能力维度（学科知识、实践技能和个人态度），这三个方面结合在一起，决定了个人的整体能力水平。

知识和技能又分为四个等级（从初级学习者到高级从业者），用来描述每个维度不同的熟练程度。态度也可以进一步划分，用来描述追求卓越、相互尊重环境的行为和思维方式，从而实现长期可持续的能力建设。详情见"2. 能力框架"部分。

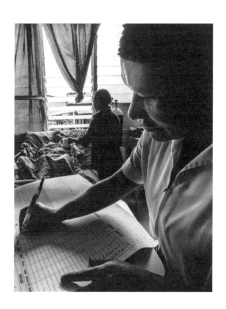

2. The Competency Framework

2. 能力框架

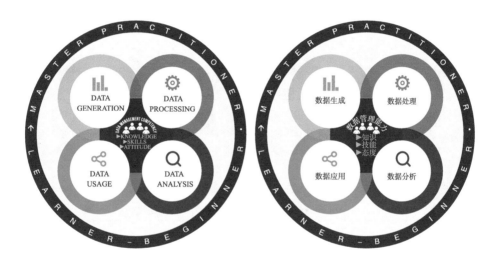

The *Data Management Competency Framework* is a practical tool to enable data management practitioners (that is line managers and HR/training managers) :

· to identify required data management role competencies and proficiency levels (required competency profile) ;

· to identify employees' current data management competencies and proficiency levels (actual competency profile) ;

· to map the gaps that exist between required and actual competency profiles; and

· to draft competency development plans at individual, team, department, division and organizational levels.

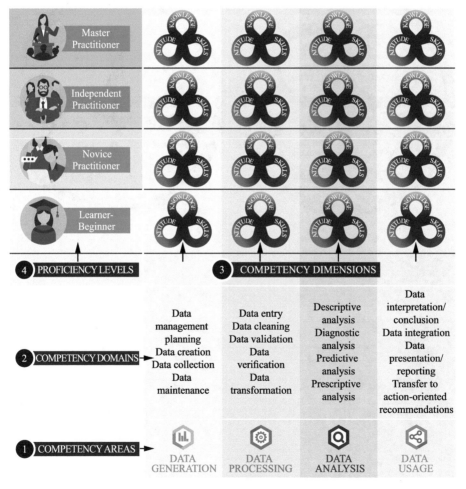

Fig. 2　Structure of the Data Management Competency Framework

《数据管理能力框架》是一个实用工具，可使数据管理人员（包括数据管理人员的直线汇报经理和人力资源/培训经理）能够：

· 确定数据管理角色所需的能力和熟练程度（需要的能力情况）。

· 确定员工当前的数据管理能力和熟练程度（实际的能力情况）。

· 确定所需能力情况与实际能力情况之间存在的差距。

· 起草个人、团队、部门和组织层面的能力发展计划。

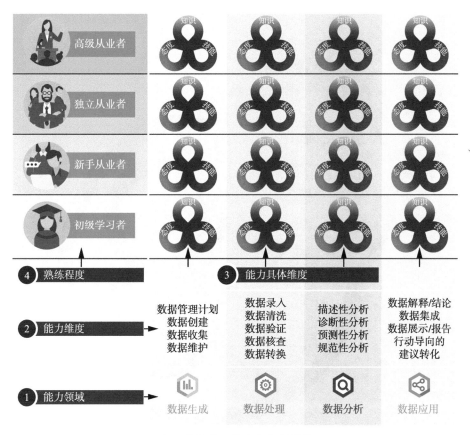

图2　数据管理能力框架的结构

The Framework is structured around four competency areas or "pillars" reflecting the four distinct stages of the data management cycle. Within each competency area are competency domains (17 in total), which are a set of distinct sub-competencies for each competency area. Within each domain, the Framework sets out the three competency dimensions (subject knowledge, practical skills and personal attitudes), which are the determinants of overall competence.

Each domain contains four designated proficiency levels (ranging from learner-beginner to master practitioner), which describe the incremental levels of proficiency by reference to a set of described technical-professional tasks that are specific, measurable and role relevant and which will determine the level of proficiency achieved by an individual employee.

■ Competency Area 1: Data Generation

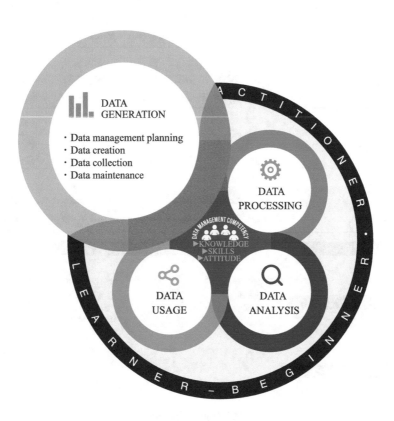

该框架围绕四个能力领域或"支柱"设计,反映了数据管理周期的四个不同阶段。每个能力领域都有能力维度(共17个),每个能力维度都有一组不同的子能力。在每个能力维度内,该框架规定了三个能力具体维度(学科知识、实践技能和个人态度),这三个能力具体维度共同决定了整体能力。

每个维度包含四个指定的熟练程度级别(从初级学习者到高级从业者),这些级别通过参考一组被清晰描述的专业技术任务来确定不同角色的熟练程度,这些任务是具体的、可测量的和与角色相关的,将决定每名员工所应达到的熟练程度。

■ 能力领域1:数据生成

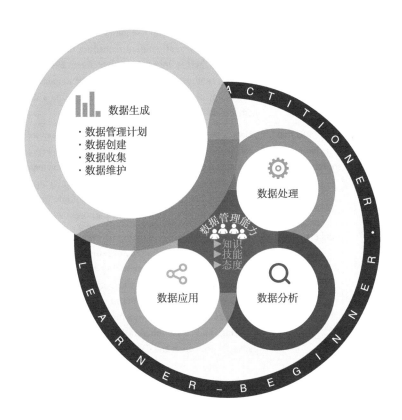

Competency domains

#		Domains	Definitions/Explanations
1		Data management planning	Data management planning is the process of delivering a formal written document (data management plan) that describes the process and methodology by which data will be created, collected and maintained throughout the life cycle of a proposed survey, trial or research activity and beyond (4-6). Factors of relevance and concern include data source identification and validation, data quality assurance and control, selection of data types (primary, secondary, tertiary), appropriate collection methodology and data maintenance (see Domain 4 below).
2		Data creation	Data creation is the process of bringing data into the realm of (human) access in an organized format for collection, analysis and interpretation (7). This can be achieved by means of quantitative and/or qualitative processes (for example, questionnaires, observational studies) and approved methods of academic and scientific enquiry and examination. In HIS, this step is normally called recording using a registry (for example, facility logbook, patient form, community health logbook) and can be done in the form of a manually prepared document or captured from the source using a data-capture device, such as a barcode reader.
3		Data collection (including sourcing)	Data collection is the process of gathering data of interest in an established systematic fashion that enables answers to be found to stated questions, to test hypotheses and to evaluate outcomes (8). Data sourcing is the process of identifying, extracting and using data from different (often multiple) internal and/or external sources to serve specific purposes (9).
4		Data maintenance	Data maintenance is concerned with setting standards for how data will be gathered, organized, stored and curated post capture and with ensuring these standards are met consistently, regardless of whether the storage is paper based or electronic (10). Data maintenance covers aspects such as organizing, coding, storing, preserving, archiving and sharing, and raises inherent issues such as data sensitivity, security protection and data integrity.

能力领域

#	领域	定义/说明
1	数据管理计划	数据管理计划是一个过程,在这个过程中需要形成一份正式的书面文件(数据管理计划)。该文件描述了拟定调查、试验或研究活动及其之后整个生命周期内数据创建、收集和维护的过程和方法[4-6]。相关因素包括数据来源的识别和验证、数据质量保证和控制、数据类型的选择(一级、二级、三级)、数据收集方法和数据维护(请参阅下面的能力领域4)
2	数据创建	数据创建是构建标准化的数据格式,并确保使用者进行收集、分析和解释的过程[7]。这可以通过定量和/或定性方法(如问卷调查、观察研究)以及获批的学术和科学询问、检查等方法来实现。在卫生信息系统(HIS)中,这一步骤通常被称为使用登记系统(例如设备日志、患者表格、社区健康日志)进行记录,并且既可以通过手动编辑文档创建,也可以通过专业数据设备(如条形码读取器)创建
3	数据收集(包括数据采集)	数据收集是以系统化方式收集所感兴趣的数据的过程,其目的是探寻答案以回答初始的问题,验证假设并评估结果[8]。数据采集是识别、提取和使用数据以满足特定目的的过程,这些数据来自不同(通常是多个)内部和/或外部来源[9]
4	数据维护	数据维护主要是为数据(纸质的、电子的)采集后的聚集、组织、存储和展示制定标准,并确保这些标准的一致性[10]。数据维护涉及获取、编码、存储、保存、归档和共享等方面的内容,并提出了数据敏感性、完整性和安全保护等内部问题

Domain 1: Data management planning

Learner-
Beginner

Knowledge Dimension

Be able to describe and explain:

· What a data management plan (or adapted term for localized use) is

· The purpose, role and importance of a data management plan in the data-generation process

· Why data are organizational assets and why data security risks should be monitored and mitigated

· The critical limitations of data

· The core International Organization for Standardization (ISO) data standards and data management planning principles

· The most common risks associated with data

· How and under what circumstances identified data risks should be escalated through the risk management structure

Skills Dimension

Be able to do the following:

· Identify any missing key information in a data request (for example, target population) and know when to seek further clarification

· Identify where ISO data standards and data management planning principles have been applied (or not) in a sample data management plan

· Categorize the levels of potential value and utilization of different data types and datasets based on the identified limitations of the data provided

· Recognize and categorize different data types and datasets in ascending order of value to the organization (D/C/B/A-low, medium, high, mission essential)

· Categorize different data types and datasets in ascending order of risk to the organization (D/C/B/A-low, medium, high, mission threatening)

维度1：数据管理计划

初级学习者

知识维度

能够描述和解释以下内容：

· 数据管理计划是什么

· 在数据生成过程中，数据管理计划的目的、角色定位和重要性

· 如何认识数据是组织资产，为什么要监测并减低数据安全风险

· 数据的主要局限性

· 国际标准化组织（ISO）的核心数据标准与数据管理计划

· 与数据相关的主要风险

· 应如何以及在何种情况下，通过应用风险管理框架及时识别更严重的数据风险

技能维度

能够做到以下几点：

· 识别数据需求中缺失的关键信息（如目标人群），并知道何时进行补充说明

· 识别在数据管理计划中应用（或不应用）ISO数据标准和数据管理计划原则的情况

· 根据所识别出的数据局限性，对不同类型数据、数据集的潜在价值和应用进行分类

· 按组织价值的升序排列，将不同类型数据和数据集进行识别和归类（D/C/B/A-低、中、高、重要）

· 按组织风险的升序排列，将不同数据类型和数据集进行识别和归类（D/C/B/A-低、中、高、重要）

Novice Practitioner

Knowledge Dimension

In addition to the Learner-Beginner knowledge, be able to describe and explain:

· The factors that influence and determine the design of data collection instruments and data presentation tools and techniques (for example, the audience, the nature of the data, whether to store in a structured or unstructured manner)

· Inherent risks within the overall data collection process

· The expected contents, structure and core elements of a data management plan (for example, the what and the how of data collection, application of the data management cycle)

· The organizational process of escalating identified data security risks

Skills Dimension

In addition to the Learner-Beginner skills, be able to do the following:

· Draft a basic data management plan based on a provided template

· Identify data risks in a provided data management plan and draft a basic risk removal/mitigation plan to address them

· Design basic data collection instruments and presentation tools and techniques

· Initiate an appropriate data security risk escalation process

Independent Practitioner

Knowledge Dimension

In addition to the Novice Practitioner knowledge, be able to describe and explain:

· Who should be involved and what technical inputs are required in drafting, reviewing and approving the data management plan including details and specifics

· The other three data generation domains with individuals specialized in these domains to create a cohesive plan

· How to map hardware, software and HR plans for a data collection exercise

· How the plan fits within the broader institutional data management vision and/or strategy

· The identified data risks and the mitigating actions in the organizational context

新手从业者

知识维度

除了初级学习者的知识外，能够描述和解释以下内容：

· 影响和决定数据收集/展示工具和技术的因素（如受众、数据的自然属性、是否以结构化的方式存储等）

· 数据收集过程中的内在风险

· 数据管理计划的内容、结构、核心要素（如数据管理周期中，数据收集和应用的内容和方式）

· 通过组织过程将已识别出的数据安全风险进行升级管理

技能维度

除了初级学习者的技能外，还要能够做到以下几点：

· 参考模板起草数据管理计划

· 识别数据管理计划中的数据风险，并起草消除/降低数据风险计划

· 设计数据收集、展示工具和技术

· 启动适当的数据风险安全升级流程

独立从业者

知识维度

除了新手从业者的知识外，还要能够描述和解释以下内容：

· 在起草、审查和授权数据管理计划（含细节）时，所涉及的人员和技术方法

· 和数据生成的另外三个维度形成一个整体方案

· 在数据收集实操中的硬件、软件和人力资源配置提供使用指南

· 数据管理计划和组织数据管理策略是如何匹配的

· 从组织的角度，识别数据风险并制定降低风险行动方案

In addition to the Novice Practitioner skills, be able to do the following:

· Set realistic goals and timelines in a data management plan

· Develop a comprehensive and realistic data management plan based on a HIS question or data demand

· Develop indicators to monitor progress as per the data management plan

· Adapt international indicators to national routine health information system(RHIS) contexts

Master Practitioner

Knowledge Dimension

In addition to the Independent Practitioner knowledge, be able to describe and explain:

· The existing data management plans in the organization and how they relate to each other

· The criteria for evaluating the effectiveness of the plan

· The data resources already available and data gaps

· The process for monitoring and evaluating the effectiveness of a data management plan

· Leadership, education and dissemination, including inputs in the areas of governance, policy and procedures design, and quality assurance of data risks

· The contingency planning process and the plan for continued data generation(for example, changing the focus of the data need and existing data generation mechanisms)in the event of a force majeure or catastrophic incident

· The policy and mechanisms for ensuring effective data governance

· How to minimize risks associated with data creation, collection and maintenance

Skills Dimension

In addition to the Independent Practitioner skills, be able to do the following:

· Foresee and anticipate future data needs

技能维度

除了新手从业者的技能外，还要能够做到以下几点：

·为数据管理计划设定目标和时间表

·基于卫生信息系统的问题或者数据需求，制定全面的数据管理计划

·为数据管理计划构建相应的监测指标体系

·将国际化的指标引入国内常规卫生信息系统（RHIS）

高级从业者

知识维度

除了独立从业者的知识外，还要能够描述和解释以下内容：

·目前各个数据管理计划及其关系

·评估数据管理计划有效性的标准

·现有数据资源的可用性及其差距

·如何监测和评估数据管理计划的有效性

·在数据风险治理、政策和过程设计、质量控制过程中的领导力、教育和传播等

·发生不可抗力或灾难性事件时，仍能够保持连续性的计划过程和数据生成过程

·确保数据治理有效的政策和机制

·如何将数据生成、收集和维护过程中的风险最小化

技能维度

除了独立从业者的技能外，还要能够做到以下几点：

·预见未来的数据需求

· Demonstrate leadership by championing and advocating for data needs and projects to gain high-level support and commitment during the data management planning process

· Critique an existing data management plan by clearly identifying areas of concern and provide solutions

· Identify and specify the resources necessary for a data management plan

· Identify roadblocks to successfully fulfilling the data request (for example, budget and HR constraints, data request too complex), and suggest alternative solutions to meet the needs of the data request

Domain 2: Data creation

Learner-Beginner

Knowledge Dimension

Be able to describe and explain:

· The differences between input, output, outcome and impact health indicators

· The concept of bias, how bias can occur and its potential effects on the dataset

· The basics of research design: types of primary research studies (for example, observational, experimental) and the key elements of each one

Skills Dimension

Be able to do the following:

· Determine which data creation method(s) is/are the most appropriate for the data request based on the pros and cons of each in context

· Appreciate different data creation methods and their suitability for different data requests

Novice Practitioner

Knowledge Dimension

In addition to the Learner-Beginner knowledge, be able to describe and explain:

· The distinctions between survey, RHIS and research data generation

· The distinct types of data (longitudinal, event, aggregate) and their use

· The different data creation methods and their application contexts for analysis and use

·在数据管理计划过程中，展示获取更高层面管理者支持的领导力

·在特定关注领域评估现有的数据管理计划，并提供改进方案

·为数据管理计划明确特定资源

·识别阻碍满足数据请求的因素（如预算和人力资源的限制、需求太复杂）并提供替代解决方案

维度2：数据创建

初级学习者

知识维度

能够描述和解释以下内容：

·不同卫生健康指标的差异：投入、产出、结果、影响

·偏倚是什么，偏倚是怎样产生的，偏倚是怎样影响数据集的

·研究设计的基础：初级研究的类型（如观察性、实验性）及其关键要素

技能维度

能够做到以下几点：

·基于数据采集的优缺点，确定最优数据采集方式

·掌握不同的数据创建方法及其能够满足的数据需求

新手从业者

知识维度

除了初级学习者的知识外，还要能够描述和解释以下内容：

·调查数据、常规卫生信息系统数据（RHIS）和研究数据之间的区别

·不同数据类型（如纵向数据、事件类型数据、汇总数据等）的区别及其应用

·不同数据创建方法及其分析和使用的应用场景

·The different data collection methods

·The relative strengths and weaknesses of each data collection method

·Awareness that some groups might be underrepresented in your dataset depending on how collection is set up

Skills Dimension

In addition to the Learner-Beginner skills, be able to do the following:

·Properly define data elements required in a relevant aggregate report or data request

·Determine and describe the key components of the data creation methods (for example, for prospective data collection, define the target population, sampling method and inclusion criteria) with moderate supervision

·Identify reliable data sources for secondary analysis (for example, national government data sources) and relevant peer-reviewed studies

·Map existing data related to the indicator to measure

·Identify whether the data required already exists and assess the feasibility of obtaining it

Independent Practitioner

Knowledge Dimension

In addition to the Novice Practitioner knowledge, be able to describe and explain:

·How data needs are identified

·The different systems available for collecting data

·The different data requirements and standards on how data should be generated and collected

·The different sampling methods available when collecting data

·The presence or existence of bias in a particular dataset

Skills Dimension

In addition to the Novice Practitioner skills, be able to do the following:

·Produce a realistic timeline for data creation (daily/monthly/quarterly/annual)

·Produce a set of indicators that are specific, measurable, achievable, relevant and time-bound

·不同的数据采集方法

·每种数据采集方法的优势与不足

·意识到因数据采集方法的不同，会导致某些群体的代表性不足

技能维度

除了初级学习者的技能外，还要能够做到以下几点：

·正确定义相关汇总报告或数据请求中所需的数据元素

·在适度的监督下，确定和描述数据创建的关键要素（如对于前瞻性数据采集需要确定的目标人群、抽样方法和纳入标准）

·为二次分析（如政府数据资源）确定合理的数据来源，检索经过相关同行评审的研究

·将需要测量的指标与现有数据进行匹配

·识别所需要的数据是否可获得

独立从业者

知识维度

除了新手从业者的知识外，还要能够描述和解释以下内容：

·如何识别数据需求

·不同系统对于数据收集的可用性

·数据产生和收集的不同需求和标准

·不同的抽样方法

·不同数据集可能存在的偏倚

技能维度

除了新手从业者的技能外，还要能够做到以下几点：

·制定可行的数据创建时间表（日/月/季度/年）

·产生一套明确的、可测量的、可完成的、有关的、具有时限性的指标

· Assess the feasibility of using one methodology over another

· Define the indicators' components to avoid any subjective interpretation of the questions

· Produce clear standard operating procedures (SOPs) for data creation, anticipating cognitive and other potential biases

Master Practitioner

Knowledge Dimension

In addition to the Independent Practitioner knowledge, be able to describe and explain:

· The main data creation activities within the organization

· What data sources are available and how they should be used for specific measurement indicators

· Potential limitations, new or upcoming changes to national and international data standards

· Potential influences and/or political barriers (for example, funding agencies, contention between departments of health units) that may impact data creation

· Situations where using specific data creation methods have failed or succeeded

· The interoperability of data collection systems

· The role and relevance of data creation in support of health policies or to monitor goals in the short and long-term

· Strategies that can be applied to minimize bias and taking a leadership role in defining and institutionalizing these strategies

Skills Dimension

In addition to the Independent Practitioner skills, be able to do the following:

· Identify a data need based on the observation and analysis of trends

· Develop a user manual explaining the data creation and how it is linked to all other components such as data processing and analysis

· Communicate an overall view of various data creations within the institution to avoid duplication or to leverage existing data creations

· Pilot and validate the developed tools for data collection

· Communicate the role and relevance of data creation in supporting health policies or in monitoring set goals in the short and long-term

·评估、选择适宜的数据收集方法

·定义指标的要素，以避免使用者对问题进行主观解释

·为数据采集制定明确的标准操作规程（SOP），预判认知偏倚和其他潜在偏倚

高级从业者

知识维度

除了独立从业者的知识外，还要能够描述和解释以下内容：

·组织内的主要数据采集活动

·哪些数据来源是可用的，以及如何用于满足特定测量指标的需求

·国家和国际的数据标准的潜在局限和未来的可能改变

·可能影响数据创建的潜在影响因素以及政策局限

·特殊的数据创建方法成败的情形

·数据采集系统的交互操作性

·数据创建在支持卫生政策或监测目标方面的短期、长期作用及相关性

·减少偏倚的策略，以及使其典型化、制度化的领导力

技能维度

除了独立从业者的技能外，还要能够做到以下几点：

·根据现况观察和趋势分析确定数据需求

·编写用户使用手册，解释数据创建过程，以及如何将其与数据处理和分析等所有其他要素关联

·在机构内传播全局性的数据创建观点，最大化使用现有数据，避免重复创建

·试行、验证已开发的数据采集工具

·交流、传播数据创建在支持卫生政策或监测目标方面的短期、长期既定目标方面的作用和相关性

·Prepare a contingency plan if data creation fails or does not achieve the initial goals

Domain 3: Data collection

Learner-
Beginner

Knowledge Dimension

Be able to describe and explain:

·The tools for routine data collection and their application in context

·Options in obtaining data and the advantages and disadvantages associated with each option

·The basics of information flow, data standards for data collection and the potential consequences of deviating from data standards

Skills Dimension

Be able to do the following:

·Encode relevant data accurately and reliably into the RHIS

·Use the digital data collection tool to do basic tasks(for example, view datasets, enter data)

·Identify data requirements and extract relevant, reliable data to suit the purpose and task

·Check, validate and verify the data source(s)

Novice
Practitioner

Knowledge Dimension

In addition to the Learner-Beginner knowledge, be able to describe and explain:

·How to identify different and reliable data sources

·Methods and standards for generating patient/client identification in digital/paper formats that can be easily authenticated and linked to existing standards, if any

·Commonly used data collection tools, techniques and methods, their advantages and disadvantages and their application contexts

Skills Dimension

In addition to the Learner-Beginner skills, be able to do the following:

·Make corrections or updates to data based on judgement

·Identify a merging ID or be able to create a merging ID

·制定数据创建失败或没有达到最初目标的应急方案、预案

维度3：数据收集

初级学习者

知识维度

能够描述和解释以下内容：

·日常数据收集工具及其应用场景

·收集数据的方法以及优劣

·基本信息流、数据收集的标准以及偏离标准的潜在影响

技能维度

能够做到以下几点：

·对常规卫生数据进行精确和可信的编码

·使用数据的管理收集工具开展基础工作（如浏览数据库、录入数据）

·识别数据需求并提取相关的可信数据去满足需求和任务

·检查、验证并核实数据来源

新手从业者

知识维度

除了初级学习者的知识外，还要能够描述和解释以下内容：

·在不同的数据来源中识别出可信的数据来源的方法

·产生电子/纸质的医生/患者主索引的方法和标准，这种方法和标准可以被验证并且和现有的标准（如果有）相一致

·常用的数据收集工具、技术和方法及其在不同应用场景下的优势和不足

技能维度

除了初级学习者的技能外，还要能够做到以下几点：

·基于专业判断修正、更新数据

·识别或创建可用于合并、链接的编码（ID）

· Break down the collected information and record it as specified in the data maintenance plan (for example, If collecting data from test results from medical records, what key data points should be collected from the lab reports and how should they be entered to fit the data element specification?) to evaluate the outcomes of the study

· Identify the format of datasets and be able to switch formats (for example, from wide to long) to suit needs and circumstances

· Implement a data collection plan as specified (for example, use their language, cultural, subject-matter knowledge/skills to conduct surveys)

· Analyse gaps in data sources and address data gaps

· Add new data to an existing dataset by creating a new case/observation, appending/binding or merging data from different sources

Independent Practitioner

Knowledge Dimension

In addition to the Novice Practitioner knowledge, be able to describe and explain:

· The relative strengths and weaknesses of each of the collection tools, techniques and methods), including the difference between paper-based and digital tools (and how they can complement each other)

· The relevant data sources for a given data collection activity or programme

· How to map the information flow related to the data for collection

· How to design data validation rules for digital tools and clear SOPs

Skills Dimension

In addition to the Novice Practitioner skills, be able to do the following:

· Design client coding systems for different data collection exercises

· Design data validation rules for digital tools and clear SOPs

· Map existing information flows related to the data to collect

·对收集到的信息进行分解，并按照数据维护计划中的规定进行记录（例如，如果希望从医疗记录中收集检验、检查结果的数据，那么需要明确应该从实验室报告中收集哪些关键数据点，并按照数据元标准输入这些数据），以评估研究结果

·识别数据集的形式并根据需求转换数据集的形式（例如，把宽的数据集转换成长的数据集）

·制定详细的数据收集计划（例如，充分考虑语言、文化、执行数据收集的知识和技能）

·分析并缩小数据需求和数据来源之间的差距

·通过输入一个新的记录/观测值或从其他来源增加/合并的方式，在现有的数据集中新增数据

独立从业者

知识维度

除了新手从业者的知识外，还要能够描述和解释以下内容：

·每种数据收集工具、技术和方法的优势和劣势，包括纸质和电子工具的差异（以及它们如何相互补充）

·给定数据收集活动或项目的相关数据源

·怎样将信息流匹配分解成可收集的数据

·如何基于数字工具和标准操作规程（SOP）设计数据验证规则

技能维度

除了新手从业者的技能外，还要能够做到以下几点：

·为不同的数据收集活动设计客户端编码系统

·基于数字工具和标准操作规程设计数据验证规则

·将信息流匹配分解成可收集的数据

· Design and develop relevant and assessor-friendly data collection tools for defined indicators

· Select relevant data collection methods for each defined indicator

· Design a set of data validation rules for digital tools

· Train assessors on data collection

· Produce or reuse standards and codes for unit of analysis (for example, client, household)

· Identify situations when the specified method may need to be modified due to context and seek approval from higher authorities, as appropriate

· Confidently launch and monitor new rounds of data collection

· Source comparable data from paper-based (logbook/tally) or digital sources

· Ascertain the data collected are fit for purpose

Master Practitioner

Knowledge Dimension

In addition to the Independent Practitioner knowledge, be able to describe and explain:

· How to design client coding systems for different data collection exercises

· The advanced coding system for data collection, including but not limited to Fast Healthcare Interoperability Resources (FHIR)

· The implied cost of data collection

· Standard requirements for international agencies such as the United States Agency for International Development and Gavi, the Vaccine Alliance

· The limitations of a selected collection system

· The potential issues with the security model of various collection systems

Skills Dimension

In addition to the Independent Practitioner skills, be able to do the following:

· Design and lead a training programme for assessors on data collection

· 为清晰界定的指标设计和开发便于评估的数据收集工具

· 为清晰界定的指标选择适当的数据收集方法

· 基于数字工具，设计一组数据验证规则

· 培训数据收集技术人员

· 基于分析单位（如客户、家庭），制定或使用已有标准编码

· 识别在哪种情况下，需要根据环境的变化修改数据收集方法，进而寻求上级的批准

· 开展并监测新一轮的数据收集进展

· 比对纸质来源和电子来源的数据

· 确定收集的数据符合研究目的

高级从业者

知识维度

除了独立从业者的知识外，还要能够描述和解释以下内容：

· 怎样对不同的数据收集项目设计客户端编码系统

· 数据收集的高级编码系统，包括但不限于快速医疗互操作性资源（FHIR）

· 数据收集的隐含成本

· 国际机构的标准要求

· 确定的数据收集系统的局限性

· 各种数据收集系统的潜在的安全问题

技能维度

除了独立从业者的技能外，还要能够做到以下几点：

· 设计并组织开展一项对于数据收集的培训

· 实际设计并开展一项数据收集活动

· Design and manage a data collection exercise in the field

· Adopt and adapt different standards in data collection as per specific areas such as international forms

· Organize user-acceptance testing of digital tools for data collection

· Seek or propose the best available market tools for data collection

Domain 4: Data maintenance

Learner-
Beginner

Knowledge Dimension

Be able to describe and explain:

· What a data maintenance plan is and its role and importance in the data-generation process

· The various and different responsibilities involved with the ownership of data

· Why and how legislation/policy may influence restrictions on data storage

· The various and differing considerations in data maintenance such as data ownership, legislative restrictions on data storage, data integrity, data retrieval, data recovery, data retention, data management responsibility, data disposal and storage cost

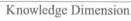

Skills Dimension

Be able to do the following:

· Outline the framework, structure or contents of a basic data maintenance plan

· Modify an existing database

· Create a basic database according to a set of given standards

Novice
Practitioner

Knowledge Dimension

In addition to the Learner-Beginner knowledge, be able to describe and explain:

· The various considerations in data storage including data ownership, legislative restrictions on data storage, data integrity, data retrieval, data recovery, data retention, data management responsibility, data disposal and storage cost

· The common database software and database management tools used in data maintenance and the pros and cons of each one

· 为数据收集的每一个环节应用不同的国际标准

· 组织对收集数据的电子工具进行用户验收

· 寻求或提出市面上最合适的数据收集工具

维度4：数据维护

初级学习者

知识维度

能够描述和解释以下内容：

· 数据维护计划及其在数据生成过程中的作用和重要性

· 与数据所有权相关的不同类别的差异化责任

· 政策法规对数据存储可能的限制和影响

· 对数据维护中不同类别的差异化责任的考量因素，如数据所有权、数据存储的政策法规限制、数据完整性、数据检索、数据恢复、数据保留、数据管理责任、数据处理和存储成本等

技能维度

能够做到以下几点：

· 提出基础数据维护计划的框架、结构或内容

· 修正现有数据库

· 根据既有的系列标准创建基础数据库

新手从业者

知识维度

除了初级学习者的知识外，还要能够描述和解释以下内容：

· 数据存储中针对包括数据所有权、数据存储的政策法规限制、数据完整性、数据检索、数据恢复、数据保留、数据管理责任、数据处理和存储成本在内的不同因素的考量

· 数据维护中常用的数据库软件、管理工具及其优缺点

Skills Dimension

In addition to the Learner-Beginner skills, be able to do the following:

· (Under guidance) apply specific treatment of the following items in the plan-data ownership and/or structure and organization, legislative restrictions, data integrity, data retrieval, data recovery, data retention, data management responsibility, data disposal and storage cost

· Create a basic database using common software packages

· Apply common database management tools specifically for use in the data maintenance processes

· Draft a template-based data maintenance plan covering, for example, the following:

■ Core structure and/or subject areas of the plan

■ Components of data architecture

Independent
Practitioner

Knowledge Dimension

In addition to the Novice Practitioner knowledge, be able to describe and explain:

· What a server is, the different server and data storing solutions available, and their advantages and disadvantages

· The technical (operational) process necessary to restore lost data from a back-up source

· The various debugging processes and solutions

· The components and standards of data architecture

· How to install different effective data security measures

Skills Dimension

In addition to the Novice Practitioner skills, be able to do the following:

· Set up a server or data-storing solutions

· Apply an authentication and security model to a database

· Maintain a database with a rigorous security model

· Resolve identified issues with the data maintenance model in place

· Use one or more data management tools/software to a basic level of proficiency

· Run routine back-ups and restore back-ups

技能维度

除了初级学习者的技能外，还要能够做到以下几点：

·（根据相关指南）对计划中的以下项目进行具体处置：数据所有权和/或结构和组织、政策法规限制、数据完整性、数据检索、数据恢复、数据保留、数据管理责任、数据处理和存储成本

·使用通用软件包创建基本数据库

·使用通用数据库管理工具用于数据维护过程

·基于模板起草数据维护计划，涵盖以下内容，例如：

■ 计划的核心结构和/或主题领域

■ 数据架构的要素

独立从业者

知识维度

除了新手从业者的知识外，还要能够描述和解释以下内容：

·服务器的基础知识、不同服务器和数据存储解决方案及其优缺点

·从备份中恢复丢失数据的技术操作过程

·多种调试过程和解决方案

·数据架构的要素和标准

·配置不同的有效数据安全工具

技能维度

除了新手从业者的技能外，还要能够做到以下几点：

·建立服务器或数据存储方案

·将身份验证和安全模式应用于数据库

·严格使用安全模式维护数据库

·利用现有的数据维护模型解决已发现的问题

·基本熟练地管理、使用一个或多个数据管理工具/软件

·例行备份和恢复备份

·Activate a recovery and/or contingency plan in the event of a disaster to ensure data are not lost or data collection continues

·Identify issues with the data maintenance model in place and report/escalate identified issues to line management

Master Practitioner

Knowledge Dimension

In addition to the Independent Practitioner knowledge, be able to describe and explain:

·The factors related to each of the key focus areas: data organization, coding, storing, preserving, archiving, sharing, and data sensitivity, security, protection and integrity

·The cost components of maintaining datasets including licences and/or hidden costs and how to rationalize them

·Institutional policies on data protection, data sharing protocols and data maintenance

·The components of a comprehensive, integrated and practical disaster recovery plan that would be activated in the event of a natural or other disaster (being a formal governance document, thus requiring approval of executive management or the board-depending on the management structure of the organization)

Skills Dimension

In addition to the Independent Practitioner skills, be able to do the following:

·Evaluate if an existing database is consistent with standards, identify areas of concern and make the necessary changes

·Anticipate the potential of a cyber-hacking

·Draft a comprehensive cyber-attack preparedness plan

·Raise the standards of institutional data maintenance to levels of best international practices

·Make a database interoperable with other in-house or external databases as per data-sharing protocols

·Draft a comprehensive set of data protection policies

·在遇到突发事件时，启动数据恢复和/或应急计划以确保数据不会丢失、数据收集继续运行

·识别数据维护模型存在的问题，并将识别出的问题报告至业务负责人

高级从业者

知识维度

除了独立从业者的知识外，还要能够描述和解释以下内容：

·各关键领域相关的因素：数据组织、编码、存储、保存、归档、共享以及数据敏感性、安全性、保护和完整性

·维护数据集的成本要素，包括许可成本和/或隐性成本及其优化

·关于数据保护、数据共享协议和数据维护的机构政策

·在遇到突发事件时，启动全面、综合和实用的数据恢复计划（该计划是经上级正式批准的）

技能维度

除了独立从业者的技能外，还要能够做到以下几点：

·评估现有数据库是否符合标准，识别值得关注的领域并进行相应调整

·预测网络黑客攻击的可能性

·起草系统的网络攻击应对计划

·将机构数据维护标准提升至国际最佳实践水平

·根据数据共享协议，实现数据库与其他内部或外部数据库的互操作性

·起草系统的数据保护政策

■ Competency Area 2: Data Processing

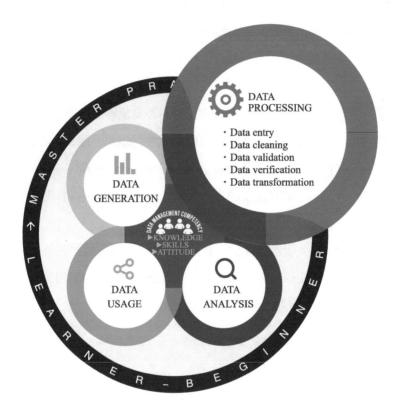

Competency domains

#		Domains	Definition
1		Data entry	Data entry is the mechanical process of direct entry and/or transcribing data records (often from paper-based sources) and/or audio into a data management system by means of keyboard entry or other technological processes *(11)*.
2		Data cleaning	Data cleaning is the process of examining data to identify blemishes in datasets (for example, wrong characters, incorrect spacing and incomplete, inaccurate, incorrect, inconsistent, irrelevant or unreliable data in a dataset) and then correcting, restoring or removing the offending data prior to processing *(11)*.
3		Data validation	Data validation consists of a series of documented data tests to ensure the validity (that is relevance, appropriateness, reliability, sourcing) and suitability of the data being reviewed *(14)*.

■ 能力领域2：数据处理

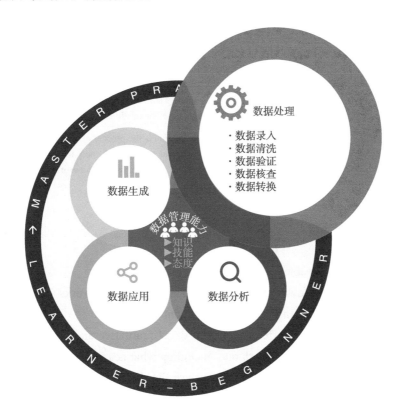

能力领域

#		领域	定义
1		数据录入	数据录入是通过键盘输入或其他技术过程进行的，将数据记录（通常是纸质来源）和/或音频直接输入或转录到数据管理系统中的技术过程[11]
2		数据清洗	数据清洗是检查数据以识别数据集中缺陷的过程（包括错误字符、不正确的空格和不完整、不准确、不正确、不一致、无关或不可靠的数据），然后对有问题的数据进行纠正、恢复或删除[11]
3		数据验证	数据验证包括一系列存档数据测试，以确保所验证数据的有效性（相关、适当、可靠和可溯源）和适用性[14]

续表

#		Domains	Definition
4		Data verification	Data verification is the process of checking data to ensure and confirm by examination and provision of objective evidence that the data being reviewed are accurate, reliable and precise to the necessary level of detail and are consistent with data quality standards expected (that is that specified requirements have been fulfilled) *(11-13)*.
5		Data transformation	Data transformation is the process of changing the format, structure or values of data with the purpose of making the data more clear, accurate, usable and useful *(10)*.

Domain 1: Data entry

Learner-Beginner

Knowledge Dimension

Be able to describe and explain:

· How a data system is structured, how it works and the role of data entry in the data management cycle

· The different types of data (qualitative and quantitative) and the subtypes of each one, including what is a variable, observation, datum/data point, and what are the different types of quantitative variables (numeric, logical, character, complex)

· The difference between a data-point value (content of field) and a label (description of that data field)

· Basic-level data-entry features and capabilities of Microsoft Excel and Word

· The definition of metadata and its function in the data management cycle (that is, the characteristics of data elements and their implications for data entry, for example, dates should be a standard format yyyymmdd, percentages should not be above 100, names should be input as text and conform to naming protocols and standards)

Skills Dimension

Be able to do the following:

· Complete basic-level data entry into the system (Excel and Word), timely, accurately and to required standards

续表

#		领域	定义
4		数据核查	数据核查是一种通过检查数据来确保并确认其准确性、可靠性和精确性的过程，通过提供客观证据来验证所审查的数据是否符合预期的数据质量标准（即满足特定的要求）[11-13]
5		数据转换	数据转换是改变数据的格式、结构或值的过程，目的是使数据更清晰、准确、可用和有价值[10]

领域1：数据录入

初级学习者

知识维度

能够描述和解释以下内容：

·数据系统的结构、运行方式以及数据录入在数据管理周期中所起的作用

·不同的数据类型（定性和定量）及其各自的子类型，包括变量、观察值、数值，以及不同变量类型（数值型、逻辑型、字符型、复杂型）

·数值（字段内容）和标签（对数据字段的描述）之间的区别

·Microsoft Excel 和 Word 的基础数据输入功能和特点

·元数据的定义及其在数据管理周期中的功能（即数据元素的特性及其对数据录入的影响，例如日期应该采用标准格式 yyyymmdd，百分比不应超过100%，姓名应以文本形式输入，并符合命名协议和标准）

技能维度

能够做到以下几点：

·及时、准确按要求标准完成基础水平（Excel 和 Word）的数据录入

· Correctly identify whether data errors are systematic or random

· Record, collect and report the data points in a logbook, tally, data entry form or any other data entry tool, accurately and within expected time frames

Novice
Practitioner

Knowledge Dimension

In addition to the Learner-Beginner knowledge, be able to describe and explain:

· The concepts of reporting completeness (timeliness, latency and consistency) and their application in data entry and data entry planning

· The most common challenges related to data entry on computer and paper-based platforms and for specific datasets (depending on the job requirements)

· The data entry flow from paper-based sources to digitalization and the implications for data entry, how to refer to original documentation to enter missing data

Skills Dimension

In addition to the Learner-Beginner skills, be able to do the following:

· Identify and overcome the most common challenges related to data entry on both digital and paper-based platforms and for specific datasets (depending on the job requirements)

· Complete a data entry flow from paper-based sources to digitalization

· Make point corrections to errors due to random chance and recognize when to escalate for assistance (for example, systemic errors that they are unable to fix)

· Identify whether the bug or fault is in the system or in the data, and dependent upon the finding, take appropriate action-for example, self-correct or escalate

· Recover "lost" or "corrupted" data and address system failure issues

· Access original documentation to enter missing data

·正确判断是系统性的还是随机的数据错误

·及时准确地通过日志簿、清单、数据输入表格或其他数据输入工具，记录、收集并报告数值

新手从业者

知识维度

除了初级学习者的知识外，能够描述和解释以下内容：

·报告完整性的概念（及时、延迟和一致），及其在数据录入和数据录入计划中的应用

·使用计算机、纸质平台或特定的数据集（根据工作要求而定）录入数据时的常见挑战

·纸质数据数字化的录入流程及其对数据录入的影响，参考原始文档补充缺失数据

技能维度

除了初级学习者的技能外，还要能够做到以下几点：

识别和克服使用计算机、纸质平台或特定的数据集（根据工作要求而定）录入数据时的常见挑战

·完成纸质数据电子化的数据录入流程

·点对点修正随机错误，识别需要上级支持的情形（例如，无法修正的系统性错误）

·识别出现问题或错误是源于系统还是数据，根据结果采取相应措施（例如，自行修正或寻求支持）

·恢复"丢失"或"损坏"的数据并解决系统故障问题

·访问原始文件以补充缺失数据

·Transfer data from the computer-assisted personal interview (CAPI) data collection system to the appropriate data management system

Independent Practitioner

Knowledge Dimension

In addition to the Novice Practitioner knowledge, be able to describe and explain:

·How to source comparable data from paper (logbook/tally) or digital sources

·How to create a template/empty database in which data are entered (structure of the dataset and explain how it is different to simple data entry)

·How to transfer stored data from the data collection software/source system to the appropriate data management system data warehouse

·The essence of potential specialty areas such as:

▪ What matrix variables are (for network data)

▪ Geographic information system (GIS) specific variables or data

▪ What CAPI data collection systems are and how data are collected and stored

Skills Dimension

In addition to the Novice Practitioner skills, be able to do the following:

·Create a template/empty database in which the data are entered (structure of the dataset)

·Complete basic tasks in potential specialty areas:

▪ Using matrix variables (for network data)

▪ Using GIS-specific variables or data

▪ Collecting and storing data using CAPI data collection systems

·Identify, report and explain problems with data entry in a manner that is standard, clear and intelligible

·Instruct junior staff and review data entry for matrices

·Transfer stored data from the data collection software/source system to the appropriate data management system data warehouse

·将计算机辅助个人访谈（CAPI）数据收集系统中的数据转移到适宜的数据管理系统中

独立从业者

知识维度

除了新手从业者的知识外，能够描述和解释以下内容：

·从纸质（日志/清单）或电子来源获取可比数据的方法

·创建一个可供输入的模板/空数据库（数据集结构与简单数据输入的区别）的方法

·将存储的数据从数据收集软件或系统中转移到适宜的数据管理系统数据仓库的方法

·潜在专业领域的关键知识，例如：

■网络数据的矩阵变量是什么

■地理信息系统（GIS）特定的变量或数据

■计算机辅助个人访谈数据收集系统是什么以及数据如何收集和存储

技能维度

除了新手从业者的技能外，还要能够做到以下几点：

·创建一个可供输入的模板/空数据库（数据集的结构）

·在潜在的专业领域完成基本任务：

■使用矩阵变量（用于网络数据）

■使用地理信息系统特定的变量或数据

■使用计算机辅助个人访谈数据收集系统进行数据的收集和存储

·以标准、清晰和可理解的方式识别、报告和解释数据输入中的问题

·指导初级员工并审核数据的输入

·将存储的数据从数据收集软件或系统中转移到适宜的数据管理系统数据仓库

· Fix systemic errors (for example, by mass dataset update) and use system tools to reduce their future occurrence (for example, data validation rules, applying correct data types)

Master Practitioner

Knowledge Dimension

In addition to the Independent Practitioner knowledge, be able to describe and explain:

· The different international standards available and used for specific datasets

· How to identify gaps and overlaps in data entry tools and correct them to streamline the data entry process

· Where and how appropriate support and direction should be provided to other practitioners

Skills Dimension

In addition to the Independent Practitioner skills, be able to do the following:

· Apply relevant international standards for specific and appropriate datasets

· Identify gaps and overlaps in data information and data entry tools

· Design data entry systems that respond to current and future data entry needs

· Train junior staff to prevent random and systemic errors using current best practice

Domain 2: Data cleaning

Learner-Beginner

Knowledge Dimension

Be able to describe and explain:

· How to identify and remove duplicates from datasets

· The rationale for and importance of recording the data cleaning process (logging data cleaning actions) including what issues have been identified and resolved

· The meanings of "error", "implausible value" and "outlier" and the differences between them conceptually

· The role and importance of data cleaning in the data management cycle

·修复系统性错误（例如，由大规模数据集更新导致的）并使用系统工具减少其未来发生的可能性（例如，数据验证规则、应用正确的数据类型）

高级从业者

知识维度

除了独立从业者的知识外，能够描述和解释以下内容：

·可用的不同国际标准及其在特定数据集的应用

·识别不同数据录入工具的功能差距和冗余，正确选用以提升数据录入效率的方法

·向其他从业者提供适当的支持和指导

技能维度

除了独立从业者的技能外，还要能够做到以下几点：

·将相关的国际标准应用于特定和适宜的数据集

·识别不同数据录入工具的功能差距和冗余

·设计符合当前和未来需求的数据录入系统

·使用目前最佳实践，培训初级员工，防止随机和系统性错误的发生

领域2：**数据清洗**

初级学习者

知识维度

能够描述和解释以下内容：

·识别和删除数据集中的重复记录的方法

·记录数据清洗过程（记录数据清洗操作）的合理性和重要性，包括记录已发现和已解决的问题

·"错误""不可信的值"和"异常值"的含义以及它们在概念上的区别

·数据清洗在数据管理周期中的角色和重要性

Be able to do the following:

· Highlight data using colours

· Format a "line list" and "pivot table"

· Identify and remove duplicates from datasets

· Identify and record "errors", recognize "implausible values" and "outliers" in a dataset, and deal with them appropriately

Novice
Practitioner

Knowledge Dimension

In addition to the Learner-Beginner knowledge, be able to describe and explain:

· The factors that influence reporting completeness (timeliness, latency and consistency) and how they are factored into the (data) cleaning process

· What diagnostic filters/screens are and how/when they are variously used in the data cleaning process

· The difference between an "error", "implausible value" and "outlier" and how to deal appropriately with each one

· Intermediate-to advanced-level data cleaning functions and capabilities in Excel and Word

· The different methods used for identification of inconsistencies in data (for example, convert data types, standardized capitalization, random white spaces, inconsistent formatting, spelling errors) and how to correct them

Skills Dimension

In addition to the Learner-Beginner skills, be able to do the following:

· Apply the various diagnostic filters/screens used in the data cleaning process

· Apply the different methods for identifying inconsistencies in data (convert data types, standardized capitalization, random white spaces, inconsistent formatting, spelling errors, etc.) and be able to correct them

· Identify data inconsistencies and identify and remove (deduplicate) datasets using different deduplication methods

技能维度

能够做到以下几点：

· 使用不同颜色突出显示数据

· 设计"行列表"和"数据透视表"

· 识别并删除数据集中的重复记录

· 识别和记录数据集中的"错误"，识别"不可信的值"和"异常值"，并进行恰当处理

新手从业者

知识维度

除了初级学习者知识外，能够描述和解释以下内容：

· 影响报告完整性（及时、延迟和一致）的因素以及如何将它们纳入（数据）清洗过程

· 诊断测试和筛选器的使用场景和使用时机的差异

· "错误""不可信的值"和"异常值"之间的区别以及如何恰当处理每种情况

· Excel 和 Word 中用于中级到高级数据清理的功能及其使用方法

· 用于识别数据不一致性的各种方法（如转换数据类型、标准化大写字母、随机空格、不一致的格式、拼写错误）以及如何修正它们

技能维度

除了初级学习者技能外，还应具备以下能力：

· 应用数据清洗过程中的各种诊断筛选器

· 应用不同的方法来识别数据中的不一致性（转换数据类型、标准化大写字母、随机空格、不一致的格式、拼写错误等），并能够进行修正

· 通过不同的去重方法，识别数据不一致性并删除（去重）数据集

· Select and use the most appropriate cleaning tools and techniques for the specific data cleaning task

· Complete data cleaning by applying the core cleaning steps/tools and using appropriate software or functions-at least District Health Information System 2 (DHIS2) /Excel, Word, if, vlookup, index-for the specific task

· Synthesize and report key data quality issues resolved

Independent Practitioner

Knowledge Dimension

In addition to the Novice Practitioner knowledge, be able to describe and explain:

· When to pass on data changes to be approved in the data (for example, delete or replace observations and data points)

· How to source and/or create diagnostic filters/screens and streamline the data cleaning process

Skills Dimension

In addition to the Novice Practitioner skills, be able to do the following:

· Source and/or create diagnostic filters/screens and streamline the data cleaning process

· Source data cleaning rules if documents are missing

· Identify and authenticate potential data errors and data outliers

· Draft a comprehensive data cleaning report

Master Practitioner

Knowledge Dimension

In addition to the Independent Practitioner knowledge, be able to describe and explain:

· How to approve changes to the data

· The features and characteristics of sensitive data

· How to anonymize datasets

· How to identify systematic and random errors in data quality and streamline the data cleaning process

Skills Dimension

In addition to the Independent Practitioner skills, be able to do the following:

·为特定的数据清洗任务选择并使用最合适的清洗工具和技术

·通过应用核心清洗步骤或工具，并使用适当的软件或功能［至少包括地区卫生信息系统2（DHIS2）/Excel，Word，if，vlookup，index］完成数据清洗

·汇总并报告已解决的关键数据质量问题

独立从业者

知识维度

除了新手从业者的知识外，还能够描述和解释以下内容：

·何时申请待批准的数据更改需求（例如，删除或替换观察值和数值）

·获取和创建诊断分类/筛选器的方式并以此优化数据清洗过程

技能维度

除了新手从业者的技能外，还能够做到以下几点：

·获取和创建诊断分类/筛选器的方式并以此优化数据清洗过程

·文档丢失情形下的数据清洗规则

·识别和验证潜在的数据错误和异常值

·起草一份系统的数据清洗报告

高级从业者

知识维度

除了独立执业者的知识外，还能够描述和解释以下内容：

·批准数据更改的方法

·敏感数据的特征和特点

·对数据集进行匿名化的方法

·识别数据中的系统性和随机错误，并优化数据清洗过程

技能维度

除了独立从业能力外，能够做到以下几点：

· Create data diagnostic filters and quality screens

· Approve changes to data (for example, delete or replace observations and data points)

· Identify sensitive data and anonymize datasets

· Identify systematic and random errors in data quality and streamline the data cleaning process

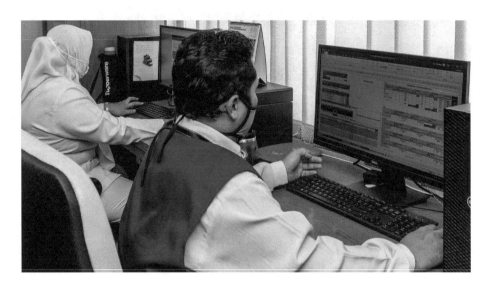

Domain 3: Data validation

Learner-Beginner

Knowledge Dimension

Be able to describe and explain:

· What data validation is and its role and importance in the data entry process

· The rules for capturing data consistently and why these rules are important

· The key characteristics used to define data quality (that is validity, accuracy, completeness, consistency, uniformity)

Skills Dimension

Be able to do the following:

· Complete basic data validation using standard rules/guidelines in place for common attributes (for example, telephone number, names, identification) and the key data quality characteristics (for example, validity, accuracy, completeness, consistency, uniformity)

· 创建数据诊断筛选器和质量筛选器

· 批准对数据的更改（例如，删除或替换观察值和数值）

· 识别敏感数据并匿名化数据集

· 识别数据中的系统性和随机性错误，并优化数据清洗过程

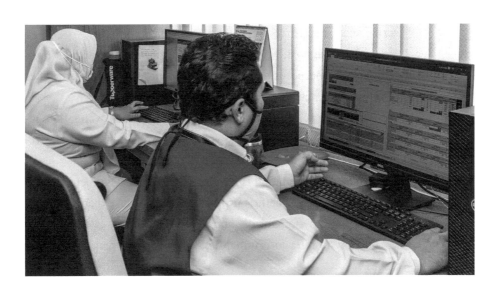

领域3：数据验证

初级学习者

知识维度

能够描述和解释以下内容：

· 数据验证是什么及其在数据录入过程中的作用和重要性

· 能够保证数据一致性的规则以及这些规则的重要性

· 用于定义数据质量的关键特征（即有效性、准确性、完整性、一致性、统一性）

技能维度

能够做到以下几点：

· 使用针对通用属性（例如，电话号码、姓名、身份信息）和关键数据质量特征（例如，有效性、准确性、完整性、一致性、统一性）的标准规则/指南完成基本的数据验证

· Document the data validation process using a standard reporting format

· Implement preliminary data validation checks as directed by senior staff

Novice
Practitioner

Knowledge Dimension

In addition to the Learner-Beginner knowledge, be able to describe and explain:

· The diagnostic tests/screens available for data validation, their specific purposes and how to use them for common attributes (for example, telephone number, names, identification)

· The purpose and rationale for recording data validation actions and how to document the validation process in a standard reporting format

· The data validation rules and diagnostic tests/screens for any type of data, their specific purposes and how to use them, comparing data points systematically and rigorously

· How to refer to original data sources to correct data quality issues

Skills Dimension

In addition to the Learner-Beginner skills, be able to do the following:

· Use diagnostic tests/screens for any type of data, comparing data points systematically and rigorously

· Revert to original data sources to correct data quality issues

· Set limits for possible numeric values for a given field and enter values that fit within a list or range of acceptable values

· Document the validation process on a standard reporting format

· Complete a data quality validation check based on the eight characteristics of data validation (originality, attribution, accuracy, consistency, legibility, contemporaneousness, endurance, completeness)

· Review source of data points (for example, paper-based documentation) to solve potential data quality issues based on the data validation findings

· Compare data points systematically and rigorously

·使用标准报告格式记录数据验证的过程

·在高级员工的指导下执行初步的数据验证检查

新手从业者

知识维度

除初级学习者所掌握的知识外，能够描述或者解释以下内容：

·数据验证中可用的诊断测试/筛选、它们的具体目的以及如何用于常见属性的验证（例如，电话号码、姓名、身份信息等）

·记录数据验证操作的目的和原理，以及如何使用标准报告格式记录验证过程

·适用于不同类型数据的验证规则和诊断测试/筛选、它们的具体目的以及使用方法，使其能够系统严谨地比较数值

·如何参考原始数据源来更正数据质量问题

技能维度

除初级学习者的技能外，能够做到以下内容：

·使用诊断测试/筛选来处理不同类型的数据，使其能够系统严谨地比较数值

·参考原始数据源来更正数据质量问题

·为特定字段设定域值范围，在域值范围内输入数值

·使用标准报告格式记录验证过程

·根据数据验证的八个特征（独创性、归属性、准确性、一致性、可读性、前瞻性、持续性、完整性）完成数据质量验证检查

·审查数值的来源（如纸质文档）以更正数据质量问题

·系统严谨地比较数值

Independent Practitioner

Knowledge Dimension

In addition to the Novice Practitioner knowledge, be able to describe and explain:

· When to approve changes in the data according to the data quality issues identified

· How to identify the difference between systematic and random errors in data quality

Skills Dimension

In addition to the Novice Practitioner skills, be able to do the following:

· Run data validation checks for any type of data

· Recognize when changes are needed and make decisions about data changes based on the data quality issues identified and on the validation findings (post-validation checks actions)

· Identify and fix systematic and random errors in data quality

· Document the post-validation checks processes on a standard reporting format

Master Practitioner

Knowledge Dimension

In addition to the Independent Practitioner knowledge, be able to describe and explain:

· The process of automating data validation tasks and streamlining the data validation process

· The steps in designing a data validation process that recognizes health, ethical and regulatory concerns

· The process of designing and running tests to identify systematic and random data quality errors

· When additional validation processes are required, and the role of data quality statements

Skills Dimension

In addition to the Independent Practitioner skills, be able to do the following:

· Automate data validation tasks and streamline the data validation process

独立从业者

知识维度

除了新手从业者所掌握的知识外，能够描述和解释以下内容：

·根据识别出的数据质量问题，确定何时批准对数据的更改

·识别数据的系统性和随机性错误的方法

技能维度

除了新手从业者所掌握的技能外，能够做到以下几点：

·对不同类型的数据进行数据验证检查

·识别是否需要变更，并根据识别到的数据质量问题和验证结果做出决策（验证后检查行动）

·识别和修复数据的系统性和随机性错误

·以标准报告格式记录验证后的检查过程

高级从业者

知识维度

除独立从业者所需掌握的知识外，能够描述或解释以下内容：

·自动化数据验证任务的过程，优化数据验证流程

·设计数据验证流程的步骤，以识别健康、伦理和法规方面所关注的关键点

·设计和运行能够识别系统性和随机性数据质量问题的测试过程

·需要额外的数据验证过程的时机，以及数据质量声明的作用

技能维度

除了独立从业者的技能外，能够做到以下几点：

·生成自动化数据验证任务，优化数据验证流程

·Create and run a data validation process that recognizes health, ethical and regulatory concerns, using appropriate data management software covering the following phases: planning, data validation, entry, (database) lock

·Design and run tests to identify systematic and random data quality errors

·Create relevant and appropriate data validation tasks

·Design and run checks to determine if changes are necessary to produce the analysis datasets either through the automated facilities of a data dictionary, or by the inclusion of explicit programme validation logic

Domain 4: Data verification

Learner-
Beginner

Knowledge Dimension

Be able to describe and explain:

·What data verification is and its role and importance in the data entry cycle

·The purpose and rationale for documenting the verification process

·The key criteria used in the data-verification process

·How to document the verification process in a standard reporting format

Skills Dimension

Be able to do the following:

·Complete verification tasks using each of the four verification methods (that is inspection, demonstration, test, analysis) under supervision

·Document the verification process on a standard reporting format

Novice
Practitioner

Knowledge Dimension

In addition to the Learner-Beginner knowledge, be able to describe and explain:

·How to migrate, merge and append data to be able to identify potential data quality issues for data verification

Skills Dimension

In addition to the Learner-Beginner skills, be able to do the following:

·Migrate, merge and append data to be able to identify poten-

·创建并运行一个数据验证流程，能够识别出健康、伦理和法规所关注的问题，并在以下阶段（计划、数据验证、录入、数据库锁定）使用适当的数据管理软件

·设计和运行能够识别系统性和随机性数据质量问题的测试

·创建相关的、恰当的数据验证任务

·设计并运行检查程序，确定是否需要通过数据字典的自动化或通过程序验证逻辑以生成分析数据集

领域4：数据核查

初级学习者

知识维度

能够描述或者解释以下内容：

·数据核查的定义，以及其在数据录入周期中的作用和重要性

·记录数据核查过程的目的和依据

·数据核查过程中使用的关键标准

·如何以标准报告格式记录数据核查过程

技能维度

能够做到以下几点：

·在指导下使用四种核查方法（即检查、演示、测试、分析）完成核查任务

·以标准报告格式记录数据核查过程

新手从业者

知识维度

除了初级学习者的知识外，能够描述和解释以下内容：

·迁移、合并和追加数据的方法，以便能够通过数据核查发现潜在的数据质量问题

技能维度

除了初级学习者的技能外，还要能够做到以下几点：

·迁移、合并和追加数据，以确定数据核查过程中可能出现

tial data quality issues for data verification

· Document the data-verification processes on a standard reporting format

Independent Practitioner

Knowledge Dimension

In addition to the Novice Practitioner knowledge, be able to describe and explain:

· What steps to take to correct potential data quality issues arising during data verification

Skills Dimension

In addition to the Learner-Beginner skills, be able to do the following:

· Correct data quality issues arising during data verification

· Design and complete both manual and/or automated data sampling and checking exercises to verify the information in the destination system matches the source system

· Use artificial intelligence and/or machine learning for data verification

· Document the post-verification checks processes on a standard reporting format

Master Practitioner

Knowledge Dimension

In addition to the Independent Practitioner knowledge, be able to describe and explain:

· How to create or adapt new best practices using current or new tools for data verification. For example, use artificial intelligence/machine learning

· How to automate data verification tasks to streamline the data verification process

Skills Dimension

In addition to the Independent Practitioner skills, be able to do the following:

· Automate data verification tasks to streamline the data verification process

· Quality control the verification activities in a data migration/merge exercise to ensure the correct transfer of data from source location

的数据质量问题

　　·以标准报告格式记录数据核查过程

独立从业者

知识维度

除了新手从业者的知识外，能够描述和解释以下内容：

　　·在数据核查过程中修正潜在的数据质量问题的方法

技能维度

除了初级学习者的技能外，还要能够做到以下几点：

　　·在数据核查过程中修正出现的数据质量问题

　　·设计并完成手动或自动化的数据抽样和检查，以验证目标系统中的信息与源系统中的信息是否匹配

　　·使用人工智能、机器学习进行数据核查

　　·以标准报告格式记录验证后的检查过程

高级从业者

知识维度

除了独立从业者的知识外，还要能够描述和解释以下内容：

　　·利用现有的新工具（例如，人工智能/机器学习）创建或调整新的最佳实践，以实现数据验证

　　·自动化数据核查任务以优化数据核查流程的方法

技能维度

除了独立从业者的技能外，还要能够做到以下几点：

　　·实现数据核查任务自动化，以优化数据核查流程

　　·在数据迁移、合并过程中对核查活动进行质量控制，确保能够正确地从源系统中传输数据

· Intervene in the recurring quality assurance process with appropriate verification intervention methodology

· Design data verification tools and/or code

· Create, adopt or adapt best practices using current or new tools for data verification

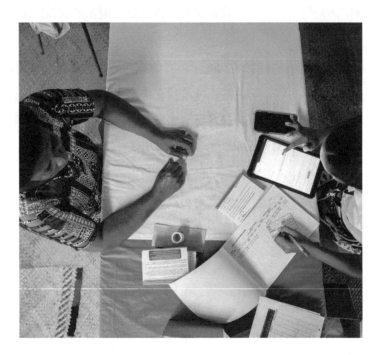

Domain 5: Data transformation

Learner-
Beginner

Knowledge Dimension

Be able to describe and explain:

· The different types of data transformation and when and how they are applied in the data transformation process

· The objective of the intended data transformation, the process required, the utility of the data elements in the dataset and how they should be combined

· The different data formats, their extraction for data generation and transformation (for example, csv, json) and how to change the data format

· The difference between a "pivot" and a "line-list" file and their implication for data transformation

・将恰当的核查干预方法应用于循环质量保证过程

・设计数据核查的工具和/或代码

・使用现有的或新的核查工具创造、应用或改进最佳实践

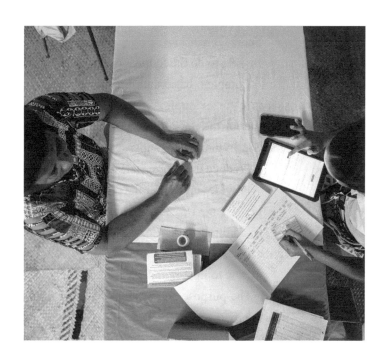

领域5：数据转换

初级学习者

知识维度

能够描述或解释以下内容：

・数据转换的不同类型及其在数据转换过程中的应用时机与场景

・数据转换的目标、数据转换的过程要求和数据元素的应用，以及三者之间如何组合使用

・不同数据的格式及其在数据生成和转换中的提取（例如，csv、json）以及数据格式的转换方法

・"数据透视表"和"行列表"文件的区别及其对数据转换的影响

·What the required data elements to process the indicator are (for example, numerator/denominator), whether the data elements are available and usable in the dataset and how they should be combined

·The purpose, benefits and challenges of data transformation

Skills Dimension

Be able to do the following:

·Complete basic data transformation tasks using appropriate software-for example, Microsoft solutions, R, Stata, Statistical Package for the Social Sciences(SPSS), statistical analysis system (SAS), Python-under supervision

·Produce the appropriate dataset for data transformation tasks

·Provide support for the creation of metadata files

Novice
Practitioner

Knowledge Dimension

In addition to the Learner-Beginner knowledge, be able to describe and explain:

·How to import and export datasets in various formats

·The purpose and rationale of documenting the data transformation process used

·How to document the transformation process in a standard reporting format

·The meanings of "unique identifier", "key variable", "data merging" and "appending/binding" and their purpose

·The different shapes of datasets(long, wide) and how to convert tabular data to row data

·How to code basic data transformations

·The difference between "data" and "metadata"

·The process of creating metadata files based on certain data transformations (for example, how an indicator was calculated)

Skills Dimension

In addition to the Learner-Beginner skills, be able to do the following:

·Import and export datasets in appropriate formats

·Complete more complex data transformation tasks, set up a clean data transformation process (for example, store working files correctly, separate raw and processed data) using Excel, with minimal

・处理指标所需的数据元素是什么（例如，分子/分母），在数据集中这些元素是否可得、可用，以及应如何组合使用

・数据转换的目的、获益和挑战

技能维度

能够做到以下几点：

・在指导下，使用恰当的软件（例如，Microsoft解决方案、R、Stata、SPSS、SAS、Python）完成基本的数据转换任务

・为数据转换任务生成恰当的数据集

・为创建元数据文件提供支持

新手从业者

知识维度

除了初级学习者的知识外，能够描述和解释以下内容：

・各种格式导入和导出数据集的方法

・数据转换过程中使用某种转换的原因及基本原理

・将转换过程记录在标准报告格式中的方法

・"唯一标识符""主键""数据合并"和"追加/绑定"的含义及目的

・数据集的不同形式（长格式、宽格式）以及如何将表格数据转换为行数据

・编写基本的数据转换代码的方法

・"数据"和"元数据"的区别

・基于特定的数据转换（例如，指标计算方式）创建元数据文件的过程

技能维度

除了初级学习者的技能外，还要能够做到以下几点：

・以适当的格式导入和导出数据集

・完成更复杂的数据转换任务，使用Excel设置简洁的数据转换流程（例如，正确存储工作文件，分离原始数据和处理后的数据），并将存储的数据从数据采集软件或系统转移到恰当的

supervision, and transfer stored data from the data collection software/source system to the appropriate data management system data warehouse (for example, extract data from DHIS2 or other platforms)

· Document the data transformation process in a standard reporting format

· Alter data formats and reshape datasets (tabular to row data and vice versa) correctly

· Code basic data transformations

· Create metadata files based on certain data transformations (for example, how an indicator was calculated)

· Merge or append/bind datasets based on unique identifiers

Independent Practitioner

Knowledge Dimension

In addition to the Novice Practitioner knowledge, be able to describe and explain:

· The difference between the extract, transform and load (ETL) and the extract, load and transform (ELT) models of data transformation and the factors that determine which transformation model is best suited to which circumstance

· The master lists in place for essential health components (for example, village, hospital) and how to use these lists in a data transformation process

· What a database management system (DBMS) is and associated data architecture, including relational and non-relational databases

· How to code advanced data transformations

· The core functions of structured query language (SQL) and other query languages

· How to recognize sensitive/confidential data and how to anonymize a dataset

Skills Dimension

In addition to the Novice Practitioner skills, be able to do the following:

· Define the objective of the intended data transformation, identify the required data elements to process the indicator (for example, numerator/denominator), identify whether the data elements are available and usable in the dataset and combine them effectively

数据管理系统中［例如，从地区卫生信息系统2（DHIS2）或其他平台提取数据］

· 以标准的报告格式记录数据转换过程

· 正确修改数据格式和调整数据集形式（表格到行数据，反之亦然）

· 编写基本的数据转换代码

· 基于特定的数据转换创建元数据文件（例如，指标计算方式）

· 基于唯一标识符合并/追加、绑定数据集

独立从业者

知识维度

除了新手从业者的知识外，能够描述和解释：

· 数据转换中提取、转换和加载（ETL）模型与提取、加载和转换（ELT）模型之间的区别，不同情况下最合适的转换模型

· 基本健康要素（例如，村庄、医院）的主列表以及如何在数据转换过程中使用这些列表

· 数据库管理系统（DBMS）及相关的数据架构，包括关系型和非关系型数据库

· 编写高级数据转换代码的方法

· 结构化查询语言（SQL）和其他查询语言的核心功能

· 识别敏感、机密数据以及如何对数据集进行匿名化处理的方法

技能维度

除了新手从业者的技能外，还要能够做到以下几点：

· 确定数据转换的预期目标，识别处理指标所需的数据元素（例如，分子/分母），以及确定在数据集中这些数据元素是否可获得、可使用，并能够有效地将其组合

·Use both ETL and ELT models of data transformation, selecting the most appropriate transformation model

·Create and use the master lists in place for essential health components (villages, hospital) in a data transformation process

·Code advanced data transformations

·Use a DBMS and associated data architecture, including relational and non-relational databases

·Use the core functions of SQL and other query languages

·Recognize sensitive/confidential data and anonymize a dataset accordingly

·Complete more advanced data transformation tasks such as "data type conversion" and "hierarchical data flattening" and complete larger-scale data-transformation tasks using scripting languages such as Python or R

Master
Practitioner

Knowledge Dimension

In addition to the Independent Practitioner knowledge, be able to describe and explain:

·How to create and/or adopt new best practices using current or new tools for data transformation (for example, design R code to automatically prepare system output data structure for further analysis)

·How to automate data transformation tasks to streamline data processing activities

Skills Dimension

In addition to the Independent Practitioner skills, be able to do the following:

·Automate data transformation tasks to streamline data processing activities

·Train junior staff on the best practice on a given software (usually Excel or SPSS for basic transformations, and Python or R for bulk transformation tasks)

·Create and/or adopt best practices using current or new tools for data transformation (for example, design R code to automatically prepare system output data structure for further analysis)

·在数据转换过程中同时使用提取、转换、加载和提取、加载和转换模型，选择最适合的转换模型

·创建并使用基本健康要素（例如，村庄、医院）的主列表，并在数据转换过程中使用

·编写高级数据转换代码

·使用数据库管理系统和相关的数据架构，包括关系型和非关系型数据库

·使用结构化查询语言和其他查询语言的核心功能

·识别敏感/涉密数据，并相应地对数据集进行匿名化处理

·完成更高级的数据转换任务，如"数据类型转换"和"层次化数据平铺"，并使用Python或R等脚本语言完成更大规模的数据转换任务

高级从业者

知识维度

除了独立从业者的知识外，能够描述和解释以下内容：

·利用现有的或者新工具开发数据转换最佳实践的方法（例如，设计R代码以自动准备系统输出数据结构以供进一步分析）

·实现数据转换任务的自动化以优化数据处理的方法

技能维度

除了独立从业者的技能外，还要能够做到以下几点：

·将数据转换任务实现自动化，以优化数据处理活动

·对初级员工进行给定软件的最佳实践培训（通常是Excel或SPSS用于基本转换，Python或R用于大规模转换任务）

·利用现有的或者新工具开发数据转换最佳实践（例如，设计R代码以自动准备系统输出数据结构以供进一步处理）

■ Competency Area 3: Data Analysis

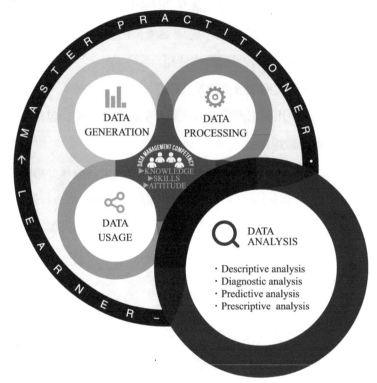

Competency domains

#		Domains	Definition
1		Descriptive analysis	Descriptive analysis is the process of using current and historical data to identify trends and relationships to provide meaningful information on current or recent events by converting raw data into a form and format that attempts to answer who, what, where and when questions *(15, 16, 18)*. Descriptive analysis is the cornerstone of data analysis and the starting point for all data insights. It may provide the first ideas about the subject of the analysis, for example, counts of the age or sex of the cohort under study.
2		Diagnostic analysis	Diagnostic analysis deals with causality and thus generates and tests hypotheses that provide crucial information about why a trend or relationship occurred. It is concerned with the search for identifying and understanding causation versus correlation, hypothesis testing, proving assumptions, etc. , such that the analysis delivers insights that are both non-obvious and value-added to the analysis process *(15, 17)*. An example could be hypothesizing and verifying whether the age or gender of the cohort under study is truly correlated with an outcome of interest.

■ 能力领域3：数据分析

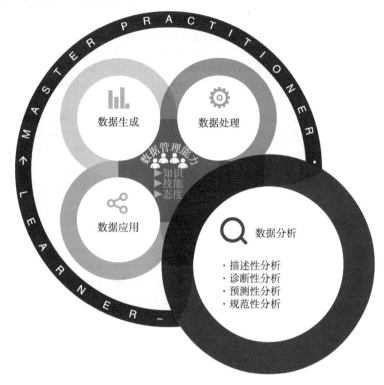

能力领域

#		领域	定义
1		描述性分析	描述性分析是使用当前和历史数据来确定趋势和关系的过程，通过将原始数据转换为试图回答谁、什么、在哪里和何时提出的问题的形式和格式，以提供有关当前或最近事件的有意义的信息[15, 16, 18]。描述性分析是数据分析的基石，也是洞察所有数据的起点。它可以提供关于分析主题的第一个想法，例如，研究队列的年龄或性别情况
2		诊断性分析	诊断性分析处理因果关系，从而生成和验证假设，这些假设提供了有关趋势或关系发生原因的关键信息。它涉及寻找识别和理解因果关系与相关性、假设检验、证明假设等，以便提供对分析过程不直观但有价值的见解[15, 17]，例如，假设和验证所研究队列的年龄或性别是否与感兴趣的结果真正相关

续表

#		Domains	Definition
3		Predictive analysis	Predictive analysis is the use of data and techniques to predict (or identify) the likelihood of future outcomes. Predictive analysis draws on past and current data and often uses comprehensive and sophisticated methods (for example, statistical algorithms and machine learning techniques) to predict the likelihood of future outcomes (15, 19). The goal is to provide a prediction of what will happen in the future. An example might be the use of age and sex as input variables to a model that calculates the likelihood of purchase behaviour to increase accuracy.
4		Prescriptive analysis	Prescriptive analysis mainly focuses on the process of using data to determine an optimal course of action. It is the most advanced, sophisticated and challenging analysis domain. Prescriptive analysis combines the outcomes from the other three analysis domains and factors in information about available resources, past and current performance, possible situations and wider environmental factors, and applies them to the process of decision-making, to assist decision-makers in determining the optimum solution from a variety of available options (15, 20). This is a complex and highly specialized type of analysis, the expertise for which is most commonly found in companies and organizations that provide specialist, third-party commercial services in this domain. An example might be the use of age and sex of all users of a social media site as input variables to an algorithm that maximizes watch-time and engagement.

Domain 1: Descriptive analysis

Learner-Beginner

Knowledge Dimension

Be able to describe and explain:

· Basic statistical concepts of central tendency (for example, average, median, mode), dispersion (for example, standard deviation) and disease frequency (for example, per cent, rate, ratio, prevalence, incidence) for the description of quantitative data

· The most appropriate choice of graph/figure (for example, bar chart, pie chart, line graph, map) for each data element or indicator, including the reasoning behind the selection

Skills Dimension

Be able to do the following:

· Identify and extract key messages and findings from a given descriptive analysis exercise

续表

#		领域	定义
3		预测性分析	预测性分析是利用数据和技术来预测（或识别）未来结果的可能性。预测性分析利用过去和当前的数据，通常使用全面而复杂的方法（如统计算法和机器学习技术）来预测未来结果的可能性[15, 19]。目标是预测未来会发生什么，如使用年龄和性别作为购买行为模型的输入变量，提高预测购买行为的准确性
4		规范性分析	规范性分析主要关注使用数据来确定最佳行动方案的过程，是最先进、最复杂、最具挑战性的分析领域。规范性分析结合了其他三个分析领域的结果和相关可用资源、过去和当前绩效、可能情况和更广泛的环境因素的信息因素，并将其应用于决策过程，以帮助决策者从各种可用选项中确定最佳解决方案[15, 20]。这是一种复杂且高度专业化的分析类型，是该领域提供专业第三方商业服务的公司和组织中最常见的专业知识，如使用社交媒体网站所有用户的年龄和性别输入变量纳入一个算法，以最大限度地提高观看时间和参与度

领域1：描述性分析

初级学习者

知识维度

能够描述或者解释以下内容：

·描述定量数据的集中趋势（例如，平均值、中位数、众数）、离散度（例如，标准差）和疾病频率（例如，百分比、率、比、患病率、发病率）的基本统计概念

·为每个数据元素或指标选择最合适的图表/图形（例如，条形图、饼图、折线图、地图）及其原因

技能维度

能够做到以下几点：

·从给定的描述性分析中识别和提取关键信息和主要发现

· Complete a basic central tendency (statistical) analysis exercise (for example, calculate average, median, mode), dispersion (for example, standard deviations), and disease frequency (for example, per cent, rate, ratio, prevalence, incidence, etc.) for description of quantitative data

· Implement content analysis, narrative interviewing and assist with the analysis from a qualitative data collection

· Complete a basic qualitative analysis exercise for a given situation using (for example, observations, textual or visual analysis of books or videos, key informant interviews and focus group discussions)

Novice
Practitioner

Knowledge Dimension

In addition to the Learner-Beginner knowledge, be able to describe and explain:

· Basic interpretations of data visualizations with one or two layers of data information (for example, rendering an indicator as three-line graphs-representing total, male and female populations-over time can highlight patterns between sexes that an aggregated graph cannot)

· Potential data quality issue, such as the concept of outliers, data quality and statistical inconsistencies, and how they affect the results of descriptive analysis

· The data elements and indicators, especially relevant key performance indicators, in a given workstation, and the correct statistical techniques to calculate them (for example, the SDG indicator for prevalence of current tobacco use should be age-standardized, the denominator of vaccination coverage should be target population and not always the entire population in country, etc.)

· The different types of statistical tables and the situations where they may be useful (for example, 2×2 table for false positivity rates)

Skills Dimension

In addition to the Learner-Beginner skills, be able to do the following:

· Create various types of statistical tables and select the situations where they may be most usefully applied (for example, 2×2 table for false positivity rates)

· 完成基本的集中趋势（统计）分析（例如，计算平均值、中位数、众数），离散趋势分析（例如，标准差）和疾病频率分析（例如，百分比、率、比、患病率、发病率）以描述定量数据

· 实施内容分析、叙述性访谈、协助对定性数据的分析

· 针对特定情形完成基本定性分析（例如，对书籍或视频进行观察性、文本性或可视化分析、关键知情人访谈和焦点小组讨论）

新手从业者

知识维度

除了初级学习者的入门知识外，还要能够描述和解释以下内容：

· 对一维或者二维数据信息的可视化结果进行基本的解释（例如，将代表总人口、男性和女性人口的指标以三线图进行呈现，可以突出性别之间的差异，而汇总图则无法做到）

· 识别潜在的数据质量问题的方法，如异常值、数据质量及统计学上的不一致性，以及它们如何影响描述性分析的结果

· 给定任务中的数据元素和指标，尤其是关键绩效指标，以及正确计算这些指标的统计方法或技术［例如，应使用年龄标化计算可持续发展目标（SDG）中的当前烟草流行率，疫苗接种覆盖率的分母应该是目标人群而不是全国总人口数］

· 不同类型的统计表及其适用情况（例如，2×2 表格适用于计算假阳性率）

技能维度

除了初级学习者的技能外，还能够做到以下几点：

· 创建不同类型的统计表并选择最适合的应用（例如，2×2 表格适用于计算假阳性率）

· Select and apply the most appropriate choice of graph/figure (for example, bar chart, pie chart, line graph, map) for each data element or indicator, for a given exercise and explain the reasoning behind selection

· Complete a basic descriptive analysis task (typically collation, summarization, aggregation, structuring and organization of data using appropriate techniques, for example, summarizing using sum of counts, and weighted average for rates, drawing 2×2 tables to describe false positivity rate of screening method vs a gold standard method)

· Visualize and present findings in a logical, coherent and meaningful way, appropriate to a given case

· Select and apply the most appropriate data elements and indicators, especially relevant key performance indicators, in a given workstation, and use the correct statistical techniques to calculate them (for example, prevalence of current tobacco use should be age-standardized, denominator of vaccination coverage should be target population instead of entire population in country, etc.)

· Complete a basic data visualization task with one or two layers of data information (for example, three-line graphs to show trend of indicator over time between total, male and female populations using Excel)

· Recognize and detect data quality issues, such as outliers, data quality and statistical inconsistencies, and identify how they affect the results of a descriptive analysis process

Independent
Practitioner

Knowledge Dimension

In addition to the Novice Practitioner knowledge, be able to describe and explain:

· The software typically used at their workstation to perform descriptive analysis and how they are used (for example, DHIS2 dashboards for monitoring immunization coverage and dropout rate, Excel)

· Basic qualitative methods and the situations where they are used (for example, observations, textual or visual analysis of books or videos, key informant interviews and focus group discussions)

·针对给定的情况，为每个数据元素或指标选择最合适的图表/图形（例如，条形图、饼图、折线图、地图），并解释选择的原因

·完成基本的描述性分析任务（通常使用适当的技术对数据进行整理、汇总、聚合、结构化和组织，例如，使用总计数汇总，使用加权平均计算率，使用2×2表格描述筛查方法与金标准方法的差异以展现阳性率）

·以符合逻辑、连贯和有意义的方式，可视化呈现结果

·选择和使用给定任务中的数据元素和指标，尤其是关键绩效指标，并使用正确的统计方法或技术计算相关指标［例如，应使用年龄标化计算可持续发展目标（SDG）中的当前烟草流行率，疫苗接种覆盖率的分母应该是目标人群而不是全国总人口数］

·通过一维或者二维的数据信息完成数据的可视化（例如，通过Excel绘制三线图，呈现代表总人口、男性和女性人口指标的时间变化趋势）

·识别和检测数据质量问题，如异常值、数据质量及统计学上的不一致性，以及它们如何影响描述性分析的结果

独立从业者

知识维度

除了新手从业者的知识外，还应能够描述和解释以下内容：

·用于进行描述性分析的软件及其使用方法（例如，用于监测免疫覆盖率和漏种率的地区卫生信息系统2、Excel）

·基本的定性方法及其使用情况（例如，对书籍或视频进行观察性、文本性或可视化分析、关键知情人访谈和焦点小组讨论）

·The results of descriptive analysis correctly and accurately using the proper units, terminology, disclaimers (for example, measles coverage for the district is 90% based on available data from 10/15 health centres)

Skills Dimension

In addition to the Novice Practitioner skills, be able to do the following:

·Perform descriptive analysis using the software typically used at their workstation and demonstrate how they are used (for example, DHIS2 dashboards for monitoring immunization coverage and dropout rate, Excel, etc.)

·Identify statistical inconsistencies before, during and after analysis and perform the correct follow-up action to address them

·Assist in the creation, selection and use of analysis outputs in data-dashboards, high-level reports and other data products

·Describe the results of a descriptive analysis exercise, accurately, using the proper units, terminology, disclaimers (for example, measles coverage for the district is 90% based on available data from 10/15 health centres)

Master Practitioner

Knowledge Dimension

In addition to the Independent Practitioner knowledge, be able to describe and explain:

·Best practices for summarizing and visualizing data and indicators relevant to the workstation (for example, component bar-graphs should be used for parts of a whole, maps [animated for years] for trends over time)

·The newest features of tools/software for developing and enhancing data summarization and visualization practices

·The relevant analytical features of other statistical software such as R, Stata, SPSS, SAS, Python, etc. and their current or potential application to a workstation's activities (for example, R script for automatically downloading and cleaning of data from DHIS2, Python for rendering online visualization for dissemination)

Skills Dimension

In addition to the Independent Practitioner skills, be able to do the following:

·使用适当的单位、术语和免责声明，正确并精准地进行描述性分析的方法（例如，根据10/15个卫生中心的可用数据，该地区的麻疹免疫覆盖率为90%）

技能维度

除了新手从业者技能外，还能够做到以下几点：

·现场使用描述性分析的软件并进行演示（例如，用于监测免疫覆盖率和漏种率的地区卫生信息系统2、Excel）

·识别事前、事中、事后统计的不一致性，并采取正确的后续行动加以解决

·在数据看板、数据报告和其他数据产品中创建、选择和使用数据分析结果

·使用适当的单位、术语和免责声明，正确并精准地进行描述性分析（例如，根据10/15个卫生中心的可用数据，该地区的麻疹免疫覆盖率为90%）

高级从业者

知识维度

除了独立从业者的知识外，还应能够描述和解释以下内容：

·总结和可视化与任务相关的数据和指标的最佳实践（例如，条形构成图用于表述整体的一部分，地图用于随时间变化的演化趋势分析）

·用于开发和增强数据概述和可视化实践的工具/软件的最新功能

·统计分析软件（如R、Stata、SPSS、SAS、Python等）的分析功能及其在当前或潜在情形中的应用（例如，使用R从地区卫生信息系统2自动下载和清理数据，使用Python进行在线可视化呈现以供传播）

技能维度

除了独立从业者的技能外，还应能够做到以下几点：

· Effectively use relevant analytic features of other statistical software such as R, Stata, SPSS, SAS, Python, etc. recognizing their current or potential application to a workstation's activities (for example, R script for automatically downloading and cleaning data from DHIS2, Python for rendering online visualization for dissemination, etc.)

· Conceptualize and design data-dashboards, high-level reports and other data products appropriate for a given use case

· Apply best practices for summarizing and visualizing data and indicators relevant to the workstation (for example, component bar-graphs should be used for parts of a whole, maps [animated for years] for trends over time)

· Experiment with the newest features of tools and software to develop and enhance data summarization and visualization practices

Domain 2: Diagnostic analysis

Learner-Beginner

Knowledge Dimension

Be able to describe and explain:

· The fundamentals and basic methods of diagnostic analysis

Skills Dimension

· Not a required skill set at this level

Novice Practitioner

Knowledge Dimension

In addition to the Learner-Beginner knowledge, be able to describe and explain:

· The most suitable methods of diagnostic analysis that should be applied based on different data types, research design and analysis purpose (methods include statistical methods or other broader methods in both qualitative and quantitative areas, data visualizations, etc.)

· Basic statistical theories (such as P value, confidence interval)

Skills Dimension

Be able to do the following:

· Select the most suitable methods of diagnostic analysis, which should be applied based on data types, research design and analysis purpose. The methods include statistical methods or other broader methods in both qualitative and quantitative areas, data visualizations, etc

·有效地使用统计分析软件（如R、Stata、SPSS、SAS、Python等）的分析功能，识别其在当前或潜在的应用情形（例如，使用R从地区卫生信息系统2自动下载和清理数据，使用Python进行在线可视化呈现以供传播）

·概念化并设计特定需求的数据看板、高水平报告和其他数据产品

·应用最佳实践来总结和可视化与任务相关的数据和指标（例如，条形构成图用于表述整体的一部分，地图用于随时间变化的演化趋势分析）

·尝试使用工具和软件的最新功能来开发和增强数据概述和可视化实践

领域2：诊断性分析

初级学习者

知识维度

能够描述和解释以下内容：

·诊断分析的基础和基本方法

技能维度

·不是本级别的必备技能

新手从业者

知识维度

除初级学习者知识外，还要能够描述和解释：

·根据不同的数据类型、研究设计和分析目的，应用最合适的诊断分析方法（包括定性、定量和数据可视化领域的统计方法或其他更广泛的方法）

·基本统计理论（如P值、置信区间等）

技能维度

除了初级学习者的技能外，还要能够做到以下几点：

·根据数据类型、研究设计和分析目的，选择最合适的诊断分析方法。这些方法包括定性、定量和数据可视化领域的统计方法或其他更广泛的方法

Independent Practitioner

Knowledge Dimension

In addition to the Novice Practitioner knowledge, be able to describe and explain:

· How to identify true differences (for example, between samples and targeted population) or test hypotheses based on a univariate (for example, t-test, Chi-square test, non-parametric test)

· How and under what circumstances advanced-level data visualization techniques are used

· How advanced software is used to generate figures/graphs with multi-layer results (for example, Tableau, R, GIS)

Skills Dimension

In addition to the Novice Practitioner skills, be able to do the following:

· Identify true differences (for example, between samples and targeted population) or test hypothesis based on a univariate (such as t test, Chi-square test, non-paramedic test)

· Make correct inferences from current data to broader more general conditions *(21)*

· Apply the chosen statistical methods to a specific task and context.

Master Practitioner

Knowledge Dimension

In addition to the Independent Practitioner knowledge, be able to describe and explain:

· How to identify potential impact and risk factors, causal and non-causal relationships (probability, likelihood) based on multi-variates and multi-levels by using advanced statistical methods (for example, correlation, regression, multi-way analysis of variance [ANOVA], survival analysis)

· The various stages, steps, procedures and challenges for a given qualitative analysis task

· How to make correct inferences from advanced statistical results and how to apply these inferences to broader more general scenarios

· How and under what circumstances advanced qualitative methods are used (grounded theory, ethnography and participant observation, visual methods, classical content analysis, experience sampling techniques, rhetorical analysis)

独立从业者

知识维度

除了新手从业者的知识外，还能够描述和解释以下内容：

·识别真正的差异（例如，样本和目标人群之间的差异）或单因素假设检验的方法（例如，t检验、卡方检验、非参数检验）

·高级数据可视化技术及其适用情况

·使用高级分析软件生成具有多维结果的图表/图形的方法（例如，Tableau、R、GIS）

技能维度

除了新手从业者的技能外，还要能做到以下几点：

·识别真正的差异（例如，样本和目标人群之间的差异）或进行单因素假设检验（例如，t检验、卡方检验、非参数检验）

·基于当前数据做出正确推断并将其扩展到一般性情况[21]

·针对特定的任务环境和背景应用适宜的统计方法

高级从业者

知识维度

除独立从业者知识外，能够描述和解释以下内容：

·基于多变量和多层次的高级统计方法（例如，相关回归、多重方差分析、生存分析），识别潜在的影响和危险因素及因果关系和非因果关系（概率、似然性）

·特定定性分析任务的不同阶段、步骤、程序和挑战

·从高级统计结果中作出正确推断，以及如何将这些推断应用于更广泛和一般性场景

·高级定性方法（扎根理论、民族志方法和参与观察法、可视化方法、内容分析法、经验取样技术、修辞分析法）及其适用情况

·The newest methods and features of tools/software and their potential for improving current diagnostic analytic procedures or subject areas

Skills Dimension

In addition to the Independent Practitioner skills, be able to do the following:

·Identify potential impact and risk factors, causal and non-causal relationships (probability, likelihood) based on multi-variates and multi-levels using advanced statistical methods (for example, correlation, regression, multi-way ANOVA, survival analysis)

·Select and apply advanced qualitative methods (grounded theory, ethnography and participant observation, visual methods, classical content analysis, experience sampling techniques, rhetorical analysis)

·Make correct inferences from advanced statistical results and apply them to broader, more general scenarios

·Complete a qualitative data analysis exercise demonstrating the various stages, steps, procedures and challenges for current analysis

·Select and apply the latest methods and newest features of tools/software for better diagnostic outcomes for same/similar areas

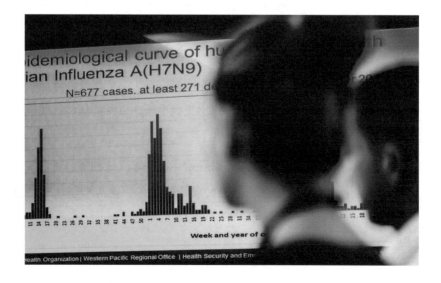

·最新的方法以及工具/软件的特色，及其对改进当前诊断分析程序或学科领域的应用价值

技能维度

除独立从业者技能外，还要能做到以下几点：

·使用多变量和多层次的高级统计方法（例如，相关回归、多重方差分析、生存分析），识别潜在的影响和危险因素及因果关系和非因果关系（概率、似然性）

·选择并应用高级定性方法（扎根理论、民族志方法和参与观察法、可视化方法、内容分析法、经验取样技术、修辞分析法）

·从高级统计结果中得出正确推论，并将其应用于更广泛、更普遍的场景

·完成定性分析任务，并展示分析的不同阶段、步骤、程序以及当前分析的挑战

·选择和应用最新方法以及工具/软件的最新功能，在相同/相似领域获得更好的诊断分析结果

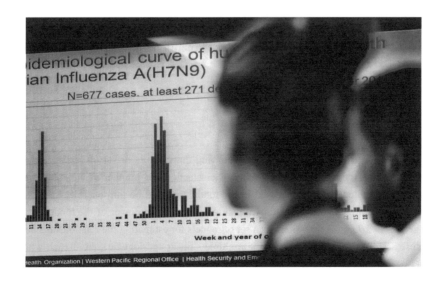

Domain 3: Predictive analysis

Learner-Beginner

Knowledge Dimension

Be able to describe and explain:

· The purpose, objective and wider context of a planned workstation analysis project and the meaning of the expected optimizations (for example, immunization unit aims to maximize immunization coverages and minimize dropout rates and vaccine vial wastage)

Skills Dimension

· Not a required skill set at this level

Novice Practitioner

Knowledge Dimension

In addition to the Learner-Beginner knowledge, be able to describe and explain:

· The concept of simple prediction and rudimentary methods for performing them (for example, extrapolating future points using arithmetic or geometric average change per year)

· The ideal qualities of a dataset (for example, selecting correct parameters/variables) for use in statistical modelling and the process of preparing these using data in a given workstation

· The general statistical principles of decision trees and regression[*] and their potential for application in predictive analysis

Skills Dimension

· Not a required skill set at this level

Independent Practitioner

Knowledge Dimension

In addition to the Novice Practitioner knowledge, be able to describe and explain:

· What longitudinal analysis is and its capability to identify data patterns and trends

---

* "Decision trees" are models for identifying the variable or set of variables that will split a dataset into the most different groups. The selection and number of variables, as well as the criteria applied for splitting used in the model, should be purposeful (for example, too many low-value variables risk compromising the predictive power of the model in a real-world setting) *(20)*. "Regression" is a set of models for estimating the relationships between variables; has different types (simple and multiple, linear and logistic, etc.) each with their own set of assumptions (main ones being normal distribution and multi-collinearity for linear and logistic regression respectively), and appropriate interpretations *(20)*.

领域3：预测性分析

初级学习者

知识维度

能够描述和解释以下内容：

·开展一项分析的目的、目标和背景，以及可预期的优化价值（例如，免疫接种的目标是最大限度地提高免疫接种覆盖率，最大限度地降低漏种率和疫苗浪费率）

技能维度

·不是本级别的必备技能

新手从业者

知识维度

除初级学习者知识外，能够描述和解释以下内容：

·简单预测的概念、方法（例如，使用算术或几何均数的年变化推断远期值）

·用于统计建模的理想数据集质量（例如，选择正确的参数/变量）及数据准备的过程

·决策树和回归*的一般统计原理及其在预测分析中的潜在应用价值

技能维度

·不是本级别的必备技能

独立从业者

知识维度

除"新手从业者"知识外，还能描述和解释以下内容：

·纵向分析及它的识别数据模式和趋势的能力

注：*"决策树"是识别变量或变量集并将变量分组的模型，该模型可将变量集划分为差异最大化亚组，应该按照明确的目标，确定纳入模型变量的选择和数量，以及变量选择标准（例如，太多的低值变量可能会降低模型的预测能力）[20]。"回归"是估计不同变量之间关系的一组模型，回归模型有不同的类型（单变量回归和多变量回归、线性回归和逻辑回归等），每一种类型都有自己的一套假设（主要的一种假设是数据基于正态分布和多元共线性的线性回归和逻辑回归），并有适当的解释[20]。

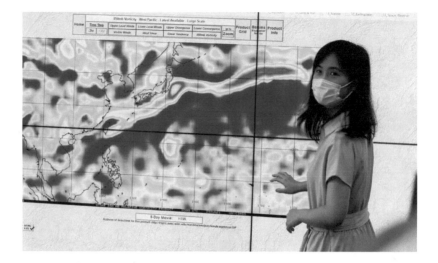

·How anomalies and/or contradictions can arise in data and how to recognize them

·The process of extrapolating to predict future outcomes while adequately communicating assumptions and limitations in the chosen analytic method

·The meanings of "linear regression", "inferential analysis", "classification" and "data segmentation"

·The basic concepts and rudimentary methods of simple predictive analysis (for example, extrapolating future points using arithmetic or geometric average change per year)

·The action points needed to design a study that will feature regression or decision trees (for example, including variables relevant to logistic regression in data collection activities to allow analysis in the future)

·The general statistical principles of predictive analysis exercises such as decision trees and regression

·The relevant datasets within a given workstation and their potential to be used for relevant predictive analyses (for example, extract regularly collected facility-based immunization database to forecast demand and avoid stockouts or wastage)

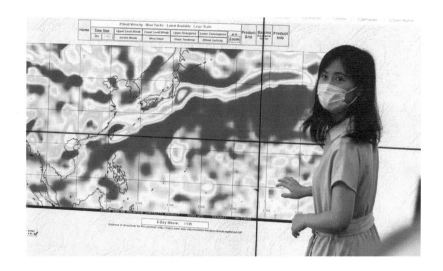

·数据出现异常和/或冲突的原因，以及如何识别

·在预测未来结果的同时，能够充分说明所选分析方法的假设和局限性

·"线性回归""推理分析""分类"和"数据分割"的含义

·简单预测分析的基本概念和基本方法（例如，使用算术或几何平均数的年变化推断远期值）

·设计研究中用于构建回归或决策树模型的关键变量（例如，在数据收集活动中纳入与逻辑回归相关的变量以便将来进行分析）

·决策树和回归等预测分析的一般统计原理

·识别可用数据集及其用于相关预测分析的能力（例如，提取定期收集的基于机构报告的免疫接种数据库，以预测需求，避免缺货或浪费）

·The value-added of different datasets to a given analysis work (for example, combining multidrug-resistant tuberculosis [MDR-TB] case dataset with health insurance database to add or verify information on co-morbidities)

·The necessary software and corresponding commands-for example, rpart. plot, integrated nested Laplace approximation (INLA) in R; pandas, numpy and matplotlib in Python-to efficiently run regression, decision trees and other analyses on relevant variables

Skills Dimension

Be able to do the following:

·Complete a predictive analysis exercise demonstrating the application of basic concepts and rudimentary methods of simple predictive analysis (for example, extrapolating future points using arithmetic or geometric average change per year)

·Select the correct parameters for a dataset for use in statistical modelling and complete the process of preparing these using data

·Carry out basic linear or logistic regression, inferential analysis, classification and data segmentation tasks

·Complete a predictive analysis exercise demonstrating the application of general statistical principles of decision trees and regression

·Select appropriate datasets and correctly apply them to a relevant predictive analysis task within a given workstation (for example, extract regularly collected facility-based immunization database to forecast demand and avoid stockouts or wastage)

·Design a study that will feature regression or decision trees (for example, incorporate child nutrition modules in periodic mother and child surveys to be able to add child weight classification as variables in logistic regression)

·Analyse past data demonstrating the capability to identify patterns and trends, while detecting anomalies and/or contradictions and extrapolate from the above to predict future outcomes while adequately communicating assumptions and limitations in the chosen analytic method

·整合不同数据集，提升特定分析的价值［例如，将耐多药结核病（MDR-TB）病例数据集与医疗保险数据库相结合，以添加或核实共病信息］

·掌握必要的软件和相应的命令，以便有效地对相关变量进行回归、决策树和其他分析［例如，R语言中的rpart.plot、集成嵌套拉普拉斯近似法（INLA）；Python语言中的pandas、numpy和matplotlib］

技能维度

能够做到以下几点：

·完成预测分析操作，展示简单预测分析的基本概念和基本方法的应用（例如，使用算术或几何平均数的年变化推断远期值）

·为用于统计建模的数据集选择正确的参数，并完成准备参数的过程

·进行基本的线性或逻辑回归、推理分析、分类和数据分割任务

·完成预测分析操作，展示应用决策树和回归的一般统计原理

·选择适当的数据集，并将其正确应用于相关预测分析（例如，提取定期收集的基于机构报告的免疫接种数据库，以预测需求，避免缺货或浪费）

·设计一项适用于回归或决策树分析的研究（例如，将儿童营养模块纳入定期母婴调查，以便在逻辑回归中将儿童体重分类作为变量）

·分析过去的数据，展示识别不同模式和发展趋势的能力，发现数据异常和/或冲突，并从上述数据中预测未来的结果，同时充分说明所选分析方法的研究假设和局限性

· Select and appropriately combine a variety of datasets to a specific analysis task(for example, combining MDR-TB case dataset with health insurance database to add or verify information on co-morbidities)

· Run accurate regression, decision trees and other analyses on relevant variables using the necessary software and corresponding commands(for example, rpart. plot, INLA in R; pandas, numpy and matplotlib in Python)

Master
Practitioner

Knowledge Dimension

In addition to the Independent Practitioner knowledge, be able to describe and explain:

· The most effective predictive analysis solutions in health context issues and viable options that can be proposed to senior management and other stakeholders

· The technical differences between variations of advanced predictive analysis techniques for a given analysis task

· The benefits, potential disadvantages, concerns and limitations of these advanced data science techniques(for example, machine learning, heuristics, neural network) for forecasting work in a given workstation

· The newest methods and features of tools/software and their potential for improving current predictive analysis procedures or subject areas

· The advantages and disadvantages of used methods and modelling techniques to guide independent and advanced practitioners to select the most appropriate one and effect proper adjustment(for example, Bayesian analysis, Poisson regression, survival analysis, time series data mining)

· The process for transferring the conceptual design of an advanced statistical model into a set of practical usable instructions to guide real-world decisions to design a notification app to warn of high-transmission area threats(for example, model for probability of infection by a particular disease, given current location and other socio-demographic factors)

·选择并正确整合各种数据集，以完成特定的分析任务（例如，将耐多药结核病病例数据集与医疗保险数据库相结合，以添加或核实有关共病的信息）

·使用必要的软件和相应的命令（例如，R语言中的rpart.plot、集成嵌套拉普拉斯近似法；Python中的pandas、numpy和matplotlib）对相关变量进行正确的回归、决策树和其他分析

高级从业者

知识维度

除了独立从业者的知识外，还能够描述和解释以下内容：

·能够向高层管理人员和其他利益相关者提出最有效的预测分析解决方案和可行的选择

·给定分析任务中高级预测分析之间的技术差异

·高级数据科学技术（例如，机器学习、启发式、神经网络）在给定预测任务中的优点、缺点、关注点和局限性

·工具/软件的最新方法和最新功能，及其在改进当前预测分析过程或专题领域中的应用潜力

·掌握分析方法和建模技术的优缺点，指导独立从业者和其他高级从业者选择最合适的方法（例如，贝叶斯分析、泊松回归、生存分析、时间序列数据分析）并进行适当调整的方法

·将高级统计模型的概念转化为可操作性的指南，用于指导真实世界的决策，进而设计一个具有提醒功能的应用程序，以警示高传播地区的风险（例如，基于当前位置和其他社会人口因素，对特定疾病感染概率进行建模）

Skills Dimension

In addition to the Independent Practitioner skills, be able to do the following:

· Select the most effective predictive analysis solutions in specific health context issues and proactively propose viable options to senior management and other stakeholders

· Select and apply the most advanced (operationally appropriate) data science techniques (for example, machine learning, heuristics, neural network) for forecasting work in a given workstation

· Select and apply the most appropriate statistical modelling* techniques in a given situation in order to understand the underlying nature of the data being analysed

· Select and apply the latest methods and newest features of tools/software for better predictive diagnostic outcomes for same/similar areas

· Select and apply the most appropriate advanced predictive analysis techniques for a given analysis work

· Select and competently apply in appropriate contexts the less commonly used methods and modelling techniques (for example, Bayesian analysis, Poisson regression, survival analysis, time series data mining) to guide independent and advanced practitioners to select the most appropriate one and effect proper adjustments

· Draft a practical users guide that translates the conceptual design of an advanced statistical model into a set of practical, usable instructions to guide real-world decisions for the design of a notification app to warn of high-transmission area threats (for example, model for probability of infection by a particular disease, given current location and other socio-demographic factors)

---

* "Statistical modelling" is a method of mathematically approximating the world. A "statistical model" is the use of statistics to build a representation of the data and then conduct analysis to infer any relationships between variables or discover insights (23). "Machine learning" is the use of mathematical and or statistical models to obtain a general understanding of the data to make predictions (24).

技能维度

除了独立从业者的技能外，还可以做到以下几点：

· 在特定的健康背景问题中选择最有效的预测分析解决方案，并向高层管理人员和其他利益相关者提出可供选择的方案

· 在给定预测任务中选择并应用高级数据科学技术（例如，机器学习、启发式、神经网络）

· 在给定情况下选择并应用最合适的统计建模技术*，以了解所分析数据的基本特征

· 选择应用最新的方法和工具/软件的功能，以便在相同/相似的领域获得更好的预测结果

· 在给定的分析任务中，选择和应用最适合的高级预测分析技术

· 完成最常用的方法和建模技术的选择，在适当的情形中充分应用（例如，贝叶斯分析、泊松回归、生存分析、时间序列数据分析），指导独立从业者和高级从业者选择最合适的方法并进行适当的调整

· 起草将高级统计模型的概念设计转化为一组实践可用的指南，以指导真实世界的决策，进而设计一个具有提醒功能的应用程序，以警示高传播地区的风险（例如，基于当前位置和其他社会人口因素，对特定疾病感染概率进行建模）

注：*"统计建模"是一种逼近真实世界的数学方法。"统计模型"是使用统计学构建数据表征，以分析推断变量间的相关性或揭示规律性[23]。"机器学习"是使用数学和/或统计模型对数据进行一般理解以进行预测的方法[24]。

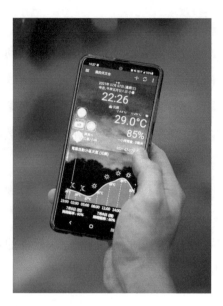

Domain 4: Prescriptive analysis

Learner-Beginner

Knowledge Dimension

Be able to describe and explain:

·The definition of prescriptive analysis especially in contrast to the other domains of data analysis

·The contexts where prescriptive analysis is used

Skills Dimension

·Not a required skill set at this level

Novice Practitioner

Knowledge Dimension

In addition to the Learner-Beginner knowledge, be able to describe and explain:

·The potential applications for data analysis (for example, useful for detecting fraud, disease, quality, safety issues patterns in real time and prescribe actions)

Skills Dimension

·Not a required skill set at this level

Independent Practitioner

Knowledge Dimension

In addition to the Novice Practitioner knowledge, be able to describe and explain:

·The basic concepts underpinning prescriptive analysis

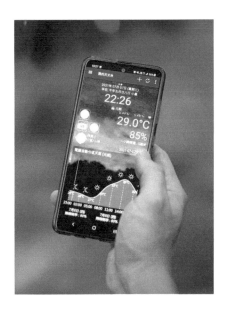

领域4：规范性分析

初级学习者

知识维度

能够描述和解释以下内容：

· 规范性分析的定义，及其与数据分析的其他领域的差异

· 规范性分析应用的场景

技能维度

· 不是本级别的必备技能

新手从业者

知识维度

除了初级学习者的知识外，还要能够描述和解释以下内容：

· 数据规范性分析的潜在应用（例如，应用于欺诈、疾病、质量、安全等问题的实时监测，并展开行动）

技能维度

· 不是本级别的必备技能

独立从业者

知识维度

除了新手从业者的知识外，还要能够描述和解释以下内容：

· 支撑规范性分析的基本概念

Skills Dimension

· Not a required skill set at this level

Master
Practitioner

Knowledge Dimension

In addition to the Independent Practitioner knowledge, be able to describe and explain:

· How to collaborate with third-party/independent companies to conduct prescriptive analysis by correctly transferring health-related needs to data language and provide health-related inputs, guidance and concerns

· How to collect and monitor the ongoing analysis related with health areas

· How to explore potential needs for prescriptive analysis in own health areas

Skills Dimension

Be able to do the following:

· Collaborate effectively with third-party/independent companies to conduct prescriptive analysis by correctly transferring health-related needs to data language, able to provide health-related inputs, guidance and concerns

· Collect and monitor the ongoing analysis related with health areas

· Explore and examine potential prescriptive analysis needs for own health areas

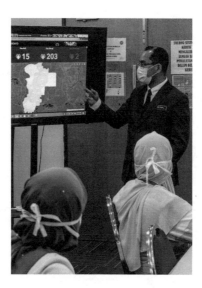

技能维度

· 不是本级别的必备技能

高级从业者

知识维度

除了独立从业者的知识外，还要能够描述和解释以下内容：

· 与第三方/独立公司合作，正确地将与健康相关的需求转化为数据语言，并提供专业支持、指导和关注，以进行规范性分析

· 收集并监控与健康领域相关的、正在开展的分析方法

· 识别本专业领域对规范性分析的潜在需求的方法

技能维度

能够做到以下几点：

· 与第三方/独立公司有效合作开展规范性分析，负责将与健康相关的需求转化为数据语言，并给予专业支持、指导和关注

· 收集并监控与健康领域相关的、正在开展的分析

· 识别、检视本专业领域对规范性分析的潜在需求

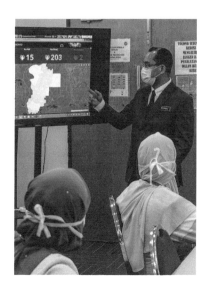

■ Competency Area 4: Data Usage

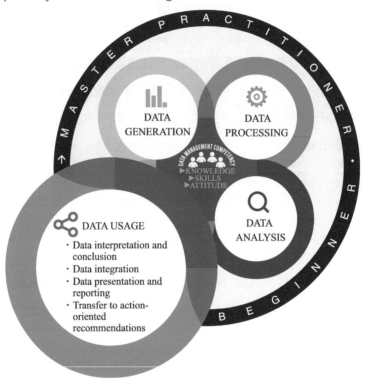

Competency domains

#		Domains	Definition
1		Data interpretation and conclusion	Data interpretation is the process of reviewing results of data analysis, making inferences, assigning meaning to the findings and producing actionable insights from which accurate and appropriate conclusions can be drawn *(25)*. Conclusion is the process of summarizing key information points and arriving at a final judgement (on an issue) based on reasoning from facts, logic and evidence of the data provided *(26, 27)*.
2		Data integration	Data integration is the process of combining data from several disparate, heterogeneous sources into a coherent data framework to retain and support a consolidated perspective of the information gathered and obtain a rounded quantitative and/ or qualitative impression of the overall effect of a particular intervention (or variable) on a defined outcome with the objective of deriving actionable insights *(9)*. Data integration can consolidate all kinds of data-structured, unstructured, batch and streaming-to do everything from basic querying of inventory databases to complex predictive analytics.

■ 能力领域4：数据应用

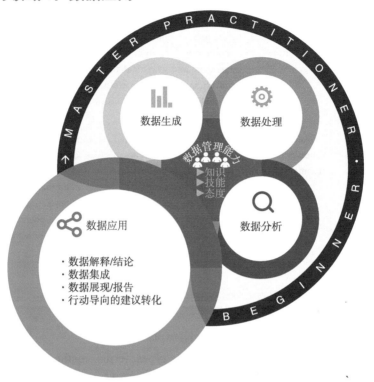

能力领域

#		领域分类	定义
1		数据解释/结论	数据解释是审查数据分析结果、做出推论、赋予研究结果意义并产生切实可行方案的过程，从中可以得出准确和适当的结论[25]。结论是根据事实、逻辑和所提供数据的证据进行推理，总结关键信息点并得出（对某个问题）最终判断的过程[26, 27]
2		数据集成	数据集成是将来自多个不同、异质性来源的数据组合成一个连贯的数据框架的过程，以保留和支持所收集信息的综合观点，并获得特定干预（或变量）对确定结果总体影响的全面定量和/或定性印象，目的是得出切实可行的方案[9]。数据集成可以整合各种类型的数据（结构化的、非结构化的、批处理的和流式的），以执行从数据库目录的基本查询到复杂的预测分析的所有操作

续表

#		Domains	Definition
3		Data presentation and reporting	Data presentation and reporting is the process of collecting unprocessed data from different sources and, by use of both narrative and graphical tools, techniques and formats, converting that data into meaningful information that provides valuable insights and enables informed decision-making (12).
4		Transfer to action-oriented recommendations	Transfer to action-oriented recommendations is the process of transferring evidence-derived knowledge into ethically sound, action-oriented recommendations (28). The focus is on the characteristics of the recommendations, which should give direction to the subsequent actions. Specific, measurable, achievable, relevant and time-bound (SMART) criteria can be used to estimate the quality of action-oriented recommendations.

Domain 1: Data interpretation and conclusion

Learner-Beginner

Knowledge Dimension

Be able to describe and explain:

·The various basic data types, terms, methods used and analysed in the results and how each method is applied in practice

·Why and how the coding (that is SAS) process (from raw data to initial results generated) is used

Skills Dimension

Be able to do the following:

·Identify the basic data types, terms, methods used and analysed in the results

·Apply each of the above (types, terms methods) in practical contexts

Novice Practitioner

Knowledge Dimension

In addition to the Learner-Beginner knowledge, be able to describe and explain:

·The meaning and application of key terms used in the process of forming conclusions (for example, inductive and deductive reasoning, premise, hypothesis, supposition, inference)

Skills Dimension

In addition to the Learner-Beginner skills, be able to do the fol-

续表

#	领域分类	定义
3	数据展现/报告	数据展现/报告是从不同来源收集未经处理的数据的过程，并通过使用叙述性和图形化工具、技术和形式，将这些数据转换为有意义的信息，从而提供有价值的方案并优化决策[12]
4	行动导向的建议转化	行动导向的建议转化是将证据知识转化为符合伦理规范的、以行动为导向的建议过程[28]。重点是建议的特征，这些特征应为后续行动指明方向。具体的、可测量的、可实现的、相关的和有时限的（SMART）标准可用于评估以行动为导向的建议的质量

领域1：数据解释/结论

初级学习者

知识维度

能够描述和解释以下内容：

·结果中使用和分析的各种基本数据类型、术语、方法以及每种方法如何在实践中应用

·使用编码（即SAS）过程（从原始数据到生成的初始结果）的原因和方式

技能维度

能够做到以下几点：

·确定结果中使用和分析的基本数据类型、术语、方法

·在实践中应用上述每一项（数据类型、术语、方法）

新手从业者

知识维度

除了初级学习者的知识外，能够描述和解释以下内容：

·形成结论过程中使用的关键术语的含义和应用（例如，归纳和演绎推理、前提、假设、推断、推理）

技能维度

除了初级学习者的技能，还要能够做到以下几点：

lowing:

· Interpret and draw basic conclusions based on the data results including data points, text, graphs, charts and maps

Independent Practitioner

Knowledge Dimension

In addition to the Novice Practitioner knowledge, be able to describe and explain:

· Advanced data types, terms, methods used and analysed in the results, how each method is applied in practice, and likely implications and consequences

· How to use data results including data points, text, graphs, charts and maps to draw accurate conclusions

Skills Dimension

In addition to the Novice Practitioner skills, be able to do the following:

· Use data results including data points, text, graphs, charts, and maps to draw accurate conclusions

· Communicate the results as applicable to different audiences

· Apply advanced data types, terms, methods used and analysed in the results, and demonstrate how each method is applied in practice

Master Practitioner

Knowledge Dimension

In addition to the Independent Practitioner knowledge, be able to describe and explain:

· The process, tools and techniques involved in "back-casting" the data resources, collection and analysis methods

· The limitations and/or restrictions of the selected process and predict potential data-gaps

· The different data resources, collection methods and distinguishing characteristics and predict potential limitations

· The key information/conclusion requirements for different types of audiences: higher-level managers for decision-making, public audiences, technical experts, field workers or lower-level implementation staff

·根据数据结果解释并得出基本结论，包括数值、文本、图表、图形和地图

独立从业者

知识维度

除了新手从业者的知识外，能够描述和解释以下内容：

·使用和分析结果的高级数据类型、术语、方法，每种方法如何在实践中应用，以及可能的含义和结果

·利用数据结果（包括数值、文本、图表、地图）得出准确的结论的方法

技能维度

除了新手从业者的技能，还要能够做到以下几点：

·使用数据结果（包括数值、文本、图表、图形和地图）得出准确的结论

·用不同受众能够接受的方式向他们传达数据的结果

·应用结果中使用的高级数据类型、术语、方法，并演示每种方法如何在实践中应用

高级从业者

知识维度

除了独立从业者的知识外，能够描述和解释以下内容：

·"回溯"数据资源、收集和分析方法所涉及的过程、工具和技术

·所选过程的限制和/或不足并预测潜在的数据差距

·不同的数据资源、采集方法和区分特征以及预测的潜在局限性

·不同类型受众的关键信息/结论要求：高层管理者、公众、技术专家、现场工作人员或基层实施人员

· From an examination of data produced, identify the specific research and analysis processes used to deliver the data, and from that, explain potential weaknesses in the selected processes that could possibly result in potentially flawed interpretations and/or conclusions

· Links with demographically similar areas that are conducting similar studies to draw a complete picture of the conclusion

· The actual and potential information gaps that will require further data collection in the next step

Skills Dimension

In addition to the Independent Practitioner skills, be able to do the following:

· Examine data produced, identify the specific research and analysis processes used to deliver the data and, from that, identify potential weaknesses in the selected processes that could possibly result in potentially flawed interpretations and/or conclusions

· Demonstrate the ability to apply the process, tools and techniques involved in data interpretation the data resources, collection, and complex analysis methods

· Identify the processes used (to deliver the data) and, from that, identify actual weaknesses in the processes that could possibly result in flawed interpretations and conclusions

· Identify potential data gaps that need further collection in future to draw further conclusions

· Compare with demographically similar health areas to extract potential lessons and identify potential information gaps that will require further collection in the next steps

· Generate and communicate key conclusions as relevant for different audience types-stakeholders: higher-level managers for decision making, public audiences, technical experts, field workers or implementation staff at the lower level

·通过对产生的数据进行检查，确定用于提供数据的具体研究和分析过程，并据此解释过程中可能导致潜在有缺陷的解释和/或结论的潜在缺陷

·和人口统计学背景相似地区的研究相关联，以得出完整的结论

·明确需要进一步收集的数据以弥合实际和潜在的信息差距

技能维度

除了独立从业者的技能，还要能够做到以下几点：

·检查生成的数据，确定具体的研究和分析过程，用于提供数据，并据此识别所选流程中可能导致潜在缺陷的解释和/或结论的潜在缺陷

·展示应用数据解释其中涉及的流程、工具和技术的能力——数据资源、收集和复杂的分析方法

·确定所使用的流程（用于传递数据），并确定实际的流程可能会导致产生不准确的解释/结论的隐患

·识别潜在的数据差距，明确未来需要进一步收集的需求，以得出进一步的结论

·与人口统计学背景相似地区的研究进行比较，提取潜在的经验，识别可能需要进一步收集的潜在信息

·生成并向不同受众类型传播相关的关键结论利益相关者：高层管理者、公众、技术专家、现场工作人员或较低级别的实施人员

Domain 2: Data integration

Learner-
Beginner

Knowledge Dimension

Be able to describe and explain：

· The core concept and principles of data integration

Skills Dimension

Be able to do the following：

· Apply the core concepts and basic principles in a basic data integration task

Novice
Practitioner

Knowledge Dimension

In addition to the Learner-Beginner knowledge, be able to describe and explain：

· How data integration processes are applied in different contexts

Skills Dimension

In addition to the Learner-Beginner skills, be able to do the following：

· Apply basic data integration processes in various integration contexts

Independent
Practitioner

Knowledge Dimension

In addition to the Novice Practitioner knowledge, be able to describe and explain：

· The importance of the data integration process in crafting the full story

· The other data requirements needed to integrate data and draw clear conclusions

· How conclusions drawn may impact routine work processes

Skills Dimension

In addition to the Novice Practitioner skills, be able to do the following：

· Integrate current findings to inform actions with the aim to improve the effectiveness of current routine work practices

Master
Practitioner

Knowledge Dimension

In addition to the Independent Practitioner knowledge, be able to describe and explain：

· What data are available from other sources and the benefit of accessing those data

领域2：数据集成

初级学习者

知识维度

能够描述和解释以下内容：

· 数据集成的核心概念和原理

技能维度

能够做到以下几点：

· 在基本数据集成任务中应用核心概念和基本原理

新手从业者

知识维度

除了初级学习者的知识外，能够描述和解释以下内容：

· 如何在不同的环境中应用数据集成流程

技能维度

除了初级学习者的技能外，还要能够做到以下内容：

· 在各种集成环境中应用基本数据集成流程

独立从业者

知识维度

除了新手从业者的知识外，能够描述和解释以下内容：

· 数据集成过程在数据应用中重要性

· 集成数据并得出明确结论所需的其他数据

· 得出的结论如何影响日常工作流程

技能维度

除了新手从业者的技能，还要能够做到以下内容：

· 整合当前的发现，为旨在提高当前日常工作有效性的干预或行动提供信息支持

高级从业者

知识维度

除了独立从业者的知识外，能够描述和解释以下内容：

· 从其他来源可以获得哪些数据以及使用这些数据的好处

·Data integration methodologies (that is data linkage and associated challenges)

·Potential limitations of not adopting integrative methods (that is data linkage)

·How to accurately draw fully informed conclusions

Skills Dimension

In addition to the Independent Practitioner skills, be able to do the following:

·Identify the different data requirements needed to integrate data and draw clear accurate conclusions

·From results/data produced, examine the quality of integration applied and from that to identify potential weaknesses that could result in flawed interpretations and conclusions

·Complete a systematic review of peer-reviewed and grey literature and present the aggregated and summarized findings from that review

·Compare multi-source data to draw accurate and fully informed conclusions

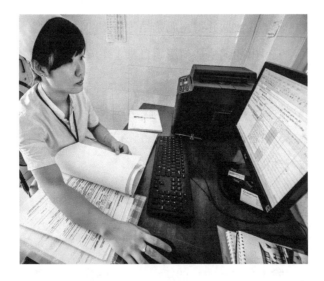

·数据集成方法（即数据链接和相关挑战）

·不采用综合方法（即数据链接和联动）的潜在局限性

·如何准确地得出全面且可靠的结论

技能维度

除了独立从业者的技能，还要能够做到以下几点：

·确定集成数据所需的不同数据要求并得出清晰准确的结论

·根据产生的结果/数据，检查集成数据的质量，并从中找出可能导致有缺陷的解释和结论的潜在问题

·完成经同行评审的论文和灰色文献的系统综述，并展示该系统综述的汇总结果和主要发现

·比较多源数据，得出全面、可靠的结论

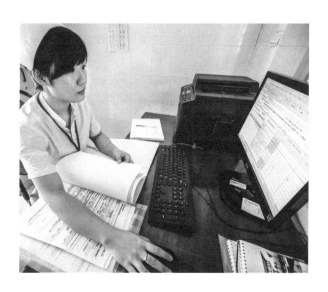

Domain 3: Data presentation and reporting

Learner-Beginner

Knowledge Dimension

Be able to describe and explain：

·The core concepts of data presentation and reporting（that is the key factors that determine the content and structure of a presentation/report-purpose, objectives, context, audience needs and expectations）, including which format, tools and techniques are most appropriate for both standard and non-standard presentations and reports

·The appropriate criteria to be used to determine the contents of a standard presentation/report

·The core principles of integrity in data reporting and how to apply them in practice

Skills Dimension

Be able to do the following：

·Identify whether the core concepts of data presentation and reporting are evident and presented in a standard report/presentation

·Identify whether core integrity principles have been applied in a particular report/presentation

·Identify whether or not the appropriate content selection criteria have been applied in a particular case

Novice Practitioner

Knowledge Dimension

In addition to the Learner-Beginner knowledge, be able to describe and explain：

·How the various content selection criteria would be applied in different standard or nonstandard presentation and reporting scenarios

Skills Dimension

In addition to the Learner-Beginner skills, be able to do the following：

·Demonstrate the practical application of content selection in different standard and nonstandard report situations

Independent Practitioner

Knowledge Dimension

In addition to the Novice Practitioner knowledge, be able to describe and explain：

·The criteria and/or principles for assessing the quality of a presentation or report

领域3：数据展示/报告

初级学习者

知识维度

能够描述和解释以下内容：

·数据展示/报告的核心概念（即决定演示/报告内容和结构的关键因素——目的、目标、背景、受众需求和期望），包括哪种格式、工具和技术最适合标准和非标准演示和报告

·用于确定标准演示/报告内容的适当标准

·数据报告完整性的核心原则以及如何在实践中应用

技能维度

能够做到以下几点：

·确定数据展示/报告的核心概念是否明显并在标准报告/演示中进行呈现

·确定在特定案例中是否应用了适当的内容选择标准

·确定在特定报告/演示文稿中是否应用了核心诚信原则

新手从业者

知识维度

除了初级学习者的知识外，能够描述和解释以下内容：

·不同的内容选择标准如何应用于不同的标准或非标准演示和报告场景

技能维度

除了初级学习者的技能，还要能够做到以下内容：

·在实际应用中，根据不同标准和非标准的报告情况选择展示内容

独立从业者

知识维度

除了新手从业者的知识外，能够描述和解释以下内容：

·评估演示或报告质量的标准和/或原则

·How to ensure data integrity in preparing and presenting data (that is recognize bias, data fabrication, manipulation, misrepresentation or falsification)

·How to examine data presentation and reporting (that is identify and explain weaknesses in the content, structure and format that could result in suboptimal understanding of the conclusions being presented)

Skills Dimension

In addition to the Novice Practitioner skills, be able to do the following:

·Apply quality assessment criteria and principles in practice to produce clear, logical and relevant structures for presentations and reports

·Select the most relevant and appropriate material to be used (and omitted) to present findings and conclusions explaining the rationale for selected material to different target audiences

·Demonstrate the use and application of data integrity principles (existence of bias, data fabrication, data manipulation, misrepresentation or falsification) in the preparation of reports and presentations

·Deliver expertly and confidently-based on thorough preparation-data integrity and subject knowledge

Master
Practitioner

Knowledge Dimension

In addition to the Independent Practitioner knowledge, be able to describe and explain:

·Data visualization tools, what they are and how they are variously used for different effects

·The key information/conclusion requirements for different types of audiences: higher-level manager for decision-making, public audiences, technical experts, field workers or implementation staff at intermediate and lower levels

Skills Dimension

In addition to the Independent Practitioner skills, be able to do the following:

·Prepare, structure and draft high-quality output in a timely manner

·如何在准备和展示数据时确保数据完整性（即识别偏倚、数据捏造、操纵、错误表述或伪造）

·如何检查数据展示/报告（即识别并解释内容、结构和格式中的缺陷，这些缺陷可能导致听众对所展示结论的理解不佳）

技能维度

除了新手从业者的技能，还要能够做到以下几点：

·应用质量评估标准和实践原则，为演示和报告提供清晰、有逻辑的以及其他相关的结构框架

·选择最相关和最合适的材料来展示调查结果和结论，向不同的目标受众解释作出上述选择的逻辑依据

·展示在准备报告和演示文稿时如何使用和应用数据的完整性原则（存在偏倚、数据捏造、数据操纵、错误表述或伪造）

·在充分准备的基础上，专业、自信地交付数据完整性分析和学科知识

高级从业者

知识维度

除了独立从业者的知识外，能够描述和解释以下内容：

·数据可视化工具，它们是什么以及它们如何以不同的方式使用，以达到不同的效果

·不同类型受众的关键信息/结论需求：高层决策管理者、公众、技术专家、现场工作人员或中下层实施人员

技能维度

除了独立从业者的技能，还要能够做到以下几点/还要能够完成以下工作/还需具备以下能力：

·及时地准备、结构化和起草高质量的展示材料

· Assess a presentation/report and identify weaknesses in the content, structure and format of the presentation/report that could result in suboptimal understanding of the conclusions being presented

· Use data visualization techniques to present data, analysis and actionable insights

· Demonstrate the presence of data integrity in the presentation of data

· Formulate and present information/conclusion requirements appropriately for different types of audiences: higher-level manager for decision-making, public audiences, technical experts, field workers or implementation staff at intermediate and lower levels

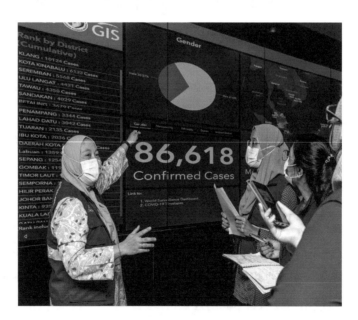

Domain 4: Transfer to action recommendations

Learner-
Beginner

Knowledge Dimension

Be able to describe and explain:

· The core concepts of how data can be used to form actionable insights such as the purpose and principles underpinning the Knowledge to Action (KTA) Framework

· Explain the meaning of each element of the SMART acronym (that is specific, measurable, achievable, relevant, time-bound)

·评估演示文稿/报告，并找出演示文稿/报告的内容、结构和格式中的缺陷，这些缺陷可能会影响对所提出结论的理解

·使用数据可视化技术来展示数据、分析和可行的观点

·证明数据展示中的数据完整性

·针对不同类型的受众（高层决策管理者、公众、技术专家、现场工作人员或中下层实施人员）制定和展示适当的信息/结论

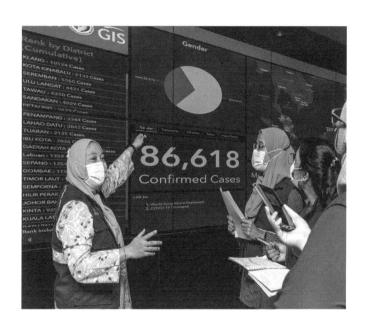

领域4：行动导向的建议转化

初级学习者

知识维度

能够描述和解释以下内容：

·如何使用数据形成可操作的核心概念，例如，支持知识到行动的目的和原则（KTA）框架

·解释SMART这个缩略词每个字母代表的含义（即特定的、可测量的、可实现的、相关的、有时限的）

Skills Dimension

Be able to do the following:

·Apply the core concepts (purpose and underpinning) principles of how data can be used to form actionable insights using the criteria of the KTA Framework

Novice
Practitioner

Knowledge Dimension

In addition to the Learner-Beginner knowledge, be able to describe and explain:

·How data are used to form actionable insights

Skills Dimension

In addition to the Learner-Beginner skills, be able to do the following:

·Apply the SMART criteria framework to the data to formulate actionable recommendations

Independent
Practitioner

Knowledge Dimension

In addition to the Novice Practitioner knowledge, be able to describe and explain:

·The purpose and principles underpinning the KTA Framework in the context of health service delivery systems, and how KTA applies to your data

·How to apply SMART criteria to research and/or recommendations

Skills Dimension

In addition to the Novice Practitioner skills, be able to do the following:

·Develop various strategies for applying actionable insights using the KTA Framework (for example, drawing on best practice examples from other KTA frameworks)

Master
Practitioner

Knowledge Dimension

In addition to the Independent Practitioner knowledge, be able to describe and explain:

·How to transition analysis to actionable insights with recommendations as an approach

·How to examine a set of KTA recommendations to identify possible weaknesses to prevent suboptimal recommendations being presented

技能维度

能够做到以下内容：

· 使用KTA框架将数据形成指导实践的可行见解的核心概念

新手从业者

知识维度

除了初级学习者的知识外，能够描述和解释以下内容：

· 如何使用数据形成可行的见解

技能维度

除了初级学习者的技能，还要能够做到以下内容：

· 将SMART标准框架应用于数据应用以制定可操作的建议

独立从业者

知识维度

除了新手从业者的知识外，能够描述和解释以下内容：

· 在卫生服务提供系统背景下的KTA框架的目的和原则，以及KTA如何应用于现有数据

· 如何将SMART标准应用于研究和/或建议

技能维度

除了新手从业者的技能，还要能够做到以下内容：

· 制定各种应用KTA框架形成可操作的见解的策略（例如，借鉴其他KTA框架的最佳实践示例）

高级从业者

知识维度

除了独立从业者的知识外，能够描述和解释以下内容：

· 如何将分析转变为可操作的概念，比如提出具体的建议的方法

· 如何检查一组KTA建议以识别可能的缺陷，以防止提出的建议不是最优的

· How to develop actionable SMART recommendations as a basis for both short and longer-term action plans for different stakeholders

· How to identify potential risks, limitations and challenges of each of the recommendations

· How data will enable future planning for activities and/or priorities in the health-care sector

· How to draw on best practice examples from other sources and to incorporate lessons from those examples to enhance current recommendations being made

Skills Dimension

In addition to the Independent Practitioner skills, be able to do the following:

· Transition analysis to actionable insights with formulation of recommendations as an approach

· Examine a set of data-insights and identify any weaknesses that could result in suboptimal recommendations being presented

· Formulate and communicate a plan for activities and/or priorities in the health-care sector

· Develop actionable (SMART) recommendations as a basis for both short and longer-term action plans for different stakeholder segments

· Draw on best-practice examples from other sources and incorporate lessons from those examples to enhance current recommendations being made

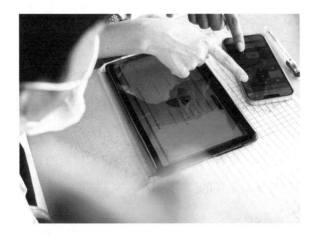

·如何制定可行的SMART建议，并作为不同利益相关者短期和长期行动计划的基础

·如何识别每项建议的潜在风险、局限性和挑战

·数据如何支持卫生系统未来活动和/或优先事项的规划

·如何借鉴其他最佳实践示例，并结合这些示例的经验教训以完善当前建议

技能维度

除了独立从业者的技能，还要能够做到以下几点：

·建立一种方法将分析转变为可行的概念，并提出建议

·检查一组数据观点并识别可能导致提出非最优建议的缺陷

·制定并传播、交流卫生系统的活动和/或优先事项的计划

·制定可行的（SMART）建议，作为不同利益相关者群体的短期和长期行动计划的基础

·借鉴其他最佳实践示例，并吸收这些示例中的经验教训，进一步完善当前建议

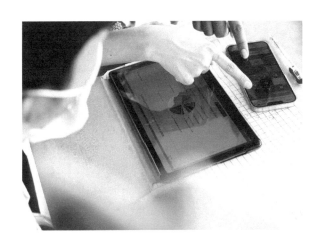

■ Attitudes

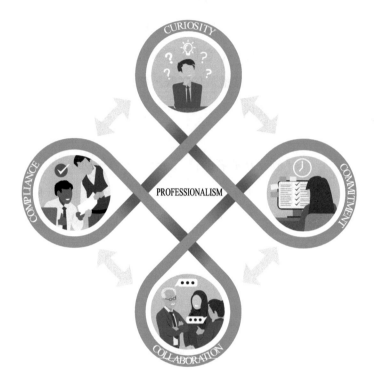

Beyond knowledge and skills, behaviours, and mindsets which create an environment characterized by unity of purpose, integrity, respect and the pursuit of excellence are essential for long-term sustainable capacity-building. The Attitudes dimension of the Framework describes four attitudinal domains which direct the behaviour of employees towards professionalism.

	Description/explanation
Professionalism	The attitudes, values, conduct and qualities that characterize or hallmark a professional person. Through their actions, professionals consistently demonstrate the qualities of competence, reliability, trustworthiness and integrity in their field of expertise. Being professional means keeping commitments, delivering high-quality work and consistently doing what it takes to demonstrate that you are a team player-being reliable, respectful and competent.

■ 态度

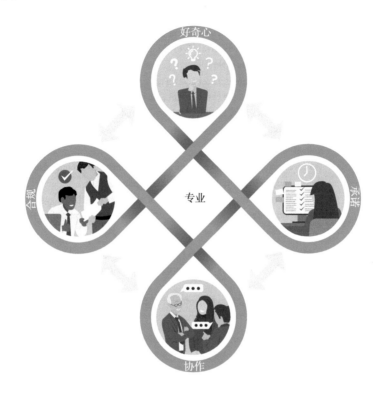

除了知识和技能之外，创造目标统一、正直、尊重和追求卓越为特征的环境的行为和心态，对于长期可持续的能力建设也至关重要。该框架的态度维度包括四个领域，这些领域引导员工的行为迈向专业化。

	定义/解释
专业精神	体现专业人士特征或标志的态度、价值观、行为和品质。专业人士通过其行动始终如一地展现出专业领域的能力、可靠性、可信度和正直品质。专业意味着信守承诺，交付高质量的工作，并始终如一、尽一切努力地证明是一名好的团队合作者——是可靠、尊重和有能力的

Domains	Demonstrated by the following observable behaviours while performing duties
Curiosity	Continuously seeks to acquire new knowledge and skills Wants to know how things work and why things happen the way they do Listens and observes attentively, questions intelligently and learns from experience and from others Open to feedback and self-reflects on actions Seeks to understand the essentials of a new task or role Demonstrates a strong appetite for learning and development Strives to refine existing or acquire new skills
Commitment	Reliable and dependable Takes responsibility for own actions and holds themself accountable for results Consistently delivers high-quality work output Perseveres to deliver results in the face of obstacles and challenges Proactively identifies ongoing professional development needs and close knowledge/skills gaps for self and others
Collaboration	Communicates and collaborates openly with colleagues and partners Displays empathic behaviour towards others, respectful of differences in cultural and beliefs of others Displays a willingness to help others in need Listens actively and questions respectfully
Compliance	Engages with colleagues and wider stakeholders in honesty, sincerity and good faith Maintains neutrality from influences and pressures Acts in the best interests of the organization Works diligently and takes pride in own work Follows company policies and complies with procedures Maintains excellent up-to-date work records, ensuring they are current, complete and accurate Maintains confidentiality and integrity Never takes advantage of position for personal gain Declares conflicts of interest, real or perceived, immediately

领域	在履行职责时表现出以下可观察到的行为
好奇心	1）不断寻求获取新知识和技能 2）想要了解事物如何运作以及事物为何以这种方式发生 3）认真倾听和观察，巧妙地提问并从经验中学习 4）乐于接受反馈并对行动进行自我反思 5）寻求了解新任务或角色的要点 6）表现出对学习和发展的强烈兴趣 7）致力于完善现有技能或获得新技能
承诺	1）可信、可靠 2）对自己的行为负责并对结果负责 3）始终如一地交付高质量的工作成果 4）面对障碍和挑战，坚持完成结果交付 5）主动识别持续的专业发展需求，并缩小自己和他人的知识/技能差距
协作	1）与同事和合作伙伴开诚布公地沟通和协作 2）对他人表现出同理心，尊重他人的文化和信仰差异 3）表现出帮助有需要的人的意愿 4）积极倾听并重视所有提问
合规	1）以诚实、真诚和善意与同事及更广泛的利益相关者交往 2）在影响和压力下保持中立 3）以组织的最佳利益为标准行事 4）勤奋工作并为自己的工作感到自豪 5）遵守机构政策程序 6）保留最新的工作记录，确保是最新的、完整的和准确的 7）保密和正直 8）绝不利用职位谋取个人利益 9）声明真实或预期的利益冲突

3. Implementation in the field

3. 实施方案

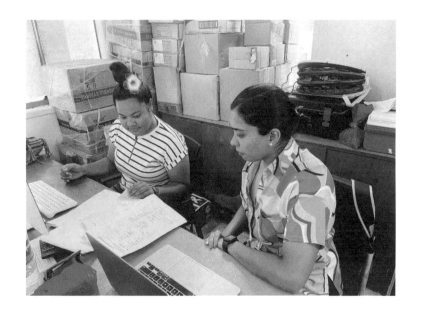

Using this *Data Management Competency Framework* comprehensively and consistently will yield a host of benefits for the HIW. The key to achieving these benefits is effective and efficient implementation and rollout of the Framework across the organization and its different levels.

In the Introduction chapter, the different target audience segments were identified. Those that are essential as "allies" for the successful adoption and rollout of the Framework were spotlighted. Local ownership of and responsibility for implementation is critical. Local management should embrace the concept and put in place the necessary oversight structures and monitoring procedures to ensure successful implementation.

To this end, it is recommended that the seven-step implementation plan (Fig. 3), which has been designed as a consequence of the testing and piloting process,

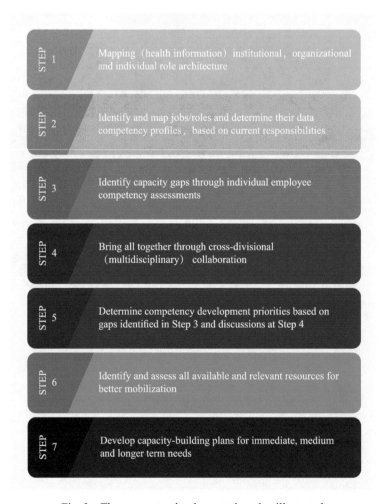

STEP 1   Mapping (health information) institutional, organizational and individual role architecture

STEP 2   Identify and map jobs/roles and determine their data competency profiles, based on current responsibilities

STEP 3   Identify capacity gaps through individual employee competency assessments

STEP 4   Bring all together through cross-divisional (multidisciplinary) collaboration

STEP 5   Determine competency development priorities based on gaps identified in Step 3 and discussions at Step 4

STEP 6   Identify and assess all available and relevant resources for better mobilization

STEP 7   Develop capacity-building plans for immediate, medium and longer term needs

Fig. 3   The seven-step implementation plan illustrated

全面一致地使用《数据管理能力框架》将为卫生信息专业人员（HIW）带来诸多益处。实现这些益处的关键是可以在组织和不同层级之间有效、高效地实施框架，并将此框架进行推广。

在引言部分，我们确定了不同的目标受众群体。那些使用和推广此框架的目标受众应得到重点关注，可以称这些人为"盟友"。本地权力和责任对框架的实施至关重要。地方管理部门应该接受这个概念，并建立必要的监督体系和监控程序，以确保框架的成功实施。

为此，建议使用在测试和试点过程中设计、形成的七步骤实施方案（图3）来指导该框架在国内的推广。同时，成员国可以根据各国国情，调整各步

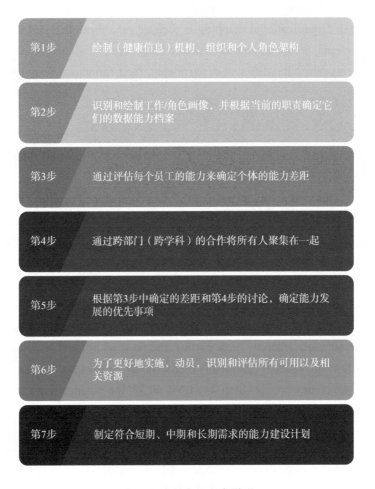

图3　七步骤实施方案说明

be used to guide in-country rollout. However, Member States may adjust the order of the steps based on the country context, such as Papua New Guinea case story on page 55.

A local, cross-departmental/divisional project management team, which should include management from the department of human resources and development, should be created to oversee and coordinate the implementation plan.

Step 1: This step involves mapping the in-country health institutions and workforce architecture. It involves three levels of mapping or analysis.

·Tier 1: Institutional mapping is focused on getting a "meta" level picture and understanding of the institutional architecture of the in-country health system-see example in Annex 3. This level involves identifying the various and different organizational entities operating within the health sector, and mapping their structures at both national and subnational levels.

·Tier 2: Organizational mapping is focused on a more detailed understanding of the internal composition and structure (organogram) of the organizations involved, documenting the different departments, their functional responsibilities, employee numbers, and the degree of engagement that the department has with health data.

·Tier 3: Individual job role mapping is focused on the employee level-identifying specific data management roles, their responsibilities and their levels of engagement with health data.

Step 2: This step involves drafting the data competency profiles. This is done by documenting the specific responsibilities of the roles and from that determining the competency areas and competency domains that are necessary to fulfil the responsibilities. Once these have been determined, the next step is to decide the level of proficiency necessary (from learner-beginner to master practitioner) to fulfil the responsibilities to a level of acceptable professional standard (see Annex 1).

Step 3: This is the gap-analysis step and involves a dialogue between employee and line manager whereby both parties discuss (and agree) the actual competency profile of the employee, which is then matched against the (predetermined) required competency profile (Step 2), from which the competency gaps will become evident and visible.

骤的顺序（如巴布亚新几内亚的案例）。

应该创建一个地方的、跨部门/分部的项目管理团队，来负责监督和协调实施计划，该团队成员应该由人力资源与发展部门的管理层等人员组成。

步骤1：这一步涉及绘制国内卫生机构和专业技术人员架构图。它包括三个层级的绘图或分析。

·层级1：机构绘图主要关注获取"元"层级的图片和对国内卫生系统的机构架构的理解——参见附件3的示例。该层级涉及确定在卫生部门内运作的各种不同组织实体，并从国家、地方两个级别上绘制其结构。

·层级2：组织绘图侧重于更详细地了解所涉及组织的内部组成和结构（组织结构图），记录不同部门、其职能职责、员工数量以及该部门与卫生数据的参与程度。

·层级3：个人工作角色绘图侧重于员工级别——确定具体的数据管理角色、责任及其与卫生数据的参与程度。

步骤2：这一步涉及起草数据能力档案。通过记录角色的具体职责来确定其必须具备的能力领域和能力维度。一旦确定了这些，下一步是决定完成职责所需的熟练程度（从初级学习者到高级从业者），以达到可接受的专业水平（附件1）。

步骤3：这是差距分析的步骤，需要员工和业务负责人之间的对话，双方讨论（并达成一致）员工的实际能力概况，然后将其与（预先确定的）所需能力概况（步骤2）进行匹配，从而明显可见出现的能力差距。

Step 4: This step involves cross-divisional collaboration whereby a cross-functional, multidisciplinary oversight team convenes to assess and evaluate the aggregated gap results and discusses these findings in the context of emerging competency gaps, strategic objectives and resources availability. This coordination team should typically consist of technical line management, the HR department and the training/development department (if separate from HR) and should be chaired by a top management representative under the coordination of a separately appointed team coordinator.

Step 5: This step is about making decisions on training/development priorities-immediate, medium and longer term-taking account of the identified competency gaps and overall strategic objectives. The key criteria for prioritizing response actions should be which competency gaps currently present the greatest risks and threats to the achievement of objectives (department, division, work unit) if left unaddressed. This does not necessarily mean the competency with the biggest gap numbers, but rather the competency gaps that present the biggest threats to achieving institutional objectives.

Step 6: This step involves a discussion on available (usually limited) resources and the most effective allocation of these resources. Resource considerations include the availability of people to lead, manage and deliver the development plan, the funding available, other (ongoing) activities within the organization that require resourcing and other planned activities and training.

Step 7: Once the priorities have been agreed and resource allocation decisions made, the final step is to draft practical and realistic development action plans to address immediate (urgent) gaps and medium-term needs. Training and development plans should be:

· Comprehensive (addressing all significant issues identified);

· Appropriate (delivering the right content to the right people);

· Consistent (applied equally, fairly and transparently); and

· Coordinated (with the right people doing the right things at the right time).

Longer-term development plans do not require detailed actions at this stage as events and priorities change over time. Nevertheless, maintaining the longer-term, sustainable capacity-building perspective is essential and should not be lost sight of. It is this "horizon focus" that provides the "north star" compass-bearing for capacity-building initiatives, which should be focused on building breadth, depth and resilience into the health information workforce over time.

步骤4：这一步涉及跨部门合作，召集一个跨职能、多学科的监督团队来评估和评价汇总的差距，并在新出现的能力差距、战略目标和资源可用性的背景下讨论这些发现。这个协调团队通常应由技术线管理层、人力资源部门和培训/发展部门（如果与人力资源分开）组成，并应在单独任命的团队协调员的协调下，由最高管理层的代表主持。

步骤5：这一步是在考虑到已确定的能力差距和整体战略目标的情况下，对培训/发展的优先事项进行决策（短期、中期和长期）。确定响应行动优先次序的关键标准应该是如果不予以解决，那么哪些能力差距将对实现目标（部门、处室、机构）造成最大风险和威胁。但这并不一定是指差距最大的能力，而是对实现机构目标影响最大的能力差距。

步骤6：这一步包括就可用资源（通常是有限的）以及对这些资源的最有效配置进行讨论。资源考虑包括领导、管理和发展计划的交付、可用的人员、资金、组织内其他需要资源支持的（正在进行的）活动以及其他计划的活动和培训。

步骤7：一旦确定了优先事项并做出资源配置的决策，最后一步就是起草实际可行的发展行动计划，以解决短期（紧急）差距和中期需求。培训和发展计划应具备以下特点：

·全面性（解决所有确定的重要问题）；

·适当性（向正确的人员提供正确的内容）；

·一致性（公平、公正和透明地应用）；

·协调性（和正确的人员在正确的时间做正确的事情）。

长期发展计划在此阶段不需要制订详细行动方案，因为其事件和优先事项会随时间变化。然而，保持较长期的、可持续的能力建设的观点是至关重要的，且不容忽视的。正是这种"视野焦点"为能力建设举措提供了方向，如"北极星"一般的存在。这些举措应着重于逐步提升卫生信息专业人员的广度、深度和韧性。

■ Case story: Papua New Guinea implementation

In order to implement its *National Health Plan 2021-2030* and associated monitoring and evaluation (M&E) plan, Papua New Guinea designed a pathway to establish an appropriately skilled HIW that could meet both current and future needs. In collaboration with WHO, Papua New Guinea commenced at Step 2 of the WHO-recommended implementation process to define the competencies of different types of health information roles: national M&E officers, provincial health information officers and medical records officers (Fig. 4). The following steps were taken:

1. Relevant job descriptions were collected and reviewed.

2. A series of interviews were conducted with different national M&E officers, provincial health information officers and medical records officers to evaluate their current roles and responsibilities as well as challenges and expectations.

3. The responsibilities of the three role types and their corresponding competencies were identified. Some critical data management domains, such as data management planning, analysis and interpretation, were not required at less advanced levels. From this analysis the draft data competency profiles were developed.

4. A two-day consultation workshop was organized by involving colleagues from the National Department of Health, including Human Resources, as well as senior management from selected Provincial Health Authorities, health information staff and development partners. The findings and draft data competency profile were reviewed, discussed and further updated.

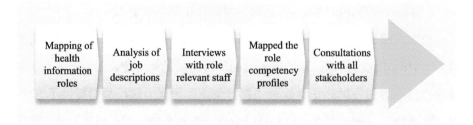

Fig. 4   The Papua New Guinea approach to developing data competency profiles for three HIW roles

■ 案例：巴布亚新几内亚的实施情况

为了实施其2021—2030年国家卫生计划及相关的监测和评估（M&E）计划，巴布亚新几内亚设计了一条路径，目的是建立一个能够满足当前和未来需求的、具备适当熟练技能的卫生信息专业人员队伍。在与世界卫生组织的合作下，巴布亚新几内亚按照世界卫生组织推荐的实施过程，从步骤2开始，来定义不同类型卫生信息角色的能力要求：国家监测评价（M&E）官员、省级卫生信息官员和病历官员（图4）。采取了以下步骤：

1. 收集、描述、审核相关职位描述。

2. 对不同的国家监测评价官员、省级卫生信息官员和病历官员进行一系列访谈，评估他们目前的角色和责任以及面临的挑战和期望。

3. 确定了三种角色类型和相应的能力要求。一些关键的数据管理领域，如数据管理计划、分析和解释，在较低级别的水平中并不需要。基于这一分析，起草了数据能力概要文件。

4. 国家卫生部门（包括人力资源）的人员以及选定的省级卫生管理局的高级管理人员、卫生信息专业人员和发展伙伴开展了为期两天的咨询研讨会。对研究结果以及起草的数据能力概要文件进行了审查、讨论和进一步的更新。

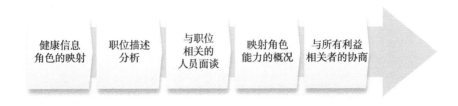

图4 巴布亚新几内亚为三类卫生信息工作者开发数据能力概要文件的方法

5. These profiles were presented for final agreement at a workshop two months later involving health information officers from all provinces and senior management from Provincial Health Authorities and the National Department of Health.

The involvement of senior management representatives in the process was critical to ensure understanding of how this work connects to broader organizational objectives, as well as for securing their commitment.

Papua New Guinea will expand the process to cover the HIW at district and health-facility levels and commence Steps 4 and 5 of the WHO procedure to develop capacity-building plans based on competency gaps measured in Step 3.

5. 这些概要文件在两个月后的研讨会上提交，供最后商定。参会人员有来自所有省份的卫生信息官员以及省级卫生管理局和国家卫生部门的高级管理人员。

高级管理人员代表参与这一进程对于确保了解这项工作如何与更广泛的组织目标相联系，同时确保他们的承诺至关重要。

巴布亚新几内亚将扩大这一工作，从而覆盖地区和卫生机构的卫生信息专业人员，并开始执行世界卫生组织推荐的程序的第4步和第5步，根据第3步中测量到的能力差距制订能力建设计划。

Annexes

附件

■ Annex 1

Indicative example of a data management competency profile

for one group of health information officers working at the provincial level

Competence Domain	Learner-Beginner	Novice Practitioner	Independent Practitioner	Master Practitioner
Data Generation				
Data management planning	X			
Data creation		X		
Data collection			X	
Data maintenance	X			
Data Processing				
Data entry			X	
Data cleaning		X		
Data validation		X		
Data verification		X		
Data transformation	X			
Data Analysis				
Descriptive analysis			X	
Diagnostic analysis		X		
Predictive analysis	X			
Prescriptive analysis	Not a required competency for this role			
Data Usage				
Data interpretation			X	
Data Integration	X			
Data reporting			X	
Transfer to action recommendations		X		

■ 附件1

数据管理能力概况示例

在省一级工作的一组卫生信息官员的数据管理能力概况示例

能力域	初级学习者	新手从业者	独立从业者	高级从业者
数据生成				
数据管理计划	X			
数据创建		X		
数据收集			X	
数据维护	X			
数据处理				
数据录入			X	
数据清洗		X		
数据验证		X		
数据核查		X		
数据转换	X			
数据分析				
描述性分析			X	
诊断性分析		X		
预测性分析	X			
规范性分析	非本职位所需的能力			
数据应用				
数据解释			X	
数据集成	X			
数据报告			X	
转向行动建议		X		

■ Annex 2

Competency (Proficiency) levels

In any professional activity there are varying degrees of competency. In this *Data Management Competency Framework*, we have categorized competency into a hierarchy of four levels ranging from learner-beginner to master practitioner as described in the table below.

Taxonomy of proficiency levels

Level	Classification	Proficiency level descriptors
1	Learner-Beginner	A graduate-level employee who has just entered the health information workforce and appointed to their first role. Has a level of theoretical knowledge and some practical experience, but this has been acquired in a "controlled-learning" college setting. Because of this, practically oriented work and task-completion experience is very limited, and the employee requires supervised, delegated, on-the-job incremental tasks with regular coaching and feedback.
2	Novice Practitioner	Has been in the role for one year or more and is developing competency across relevant role domains but continues to work under supervision and oversight on all but most basic delegated professional tasks.
3	Independent Practitioner	Is independently and reliably competent in the specific domain. Rarely is there a need to refer for advice or guidance-only in unique or exceptional situations.
4	Master Practitioner	Has achieved mastery in the domain. Is an acknowledged expert and expands the boundaries of domain knowledge through research, experimentation and innovation. Is recognized as a trainer and mentor to juniors and is sought after by peers and others for technical advice and guidance.

■ 附件2

能力（熟练程度）等级

任何专业活动都有不同程度的能力。在本《数据管理能力框架》中，我们将能力分为四个等级，从初级学习者到高级从业者，如下表所示。

熟练程度等级分类

等级	分类	熟练等级描述
1	初级学习者	刚进入医疗信息工作岗位并被任命担任第一个职务的研究生水平的员工。具有一定的理论知识和实践经验，但这些都是在"受控学习"的大学环境中获得的。因此，以实践为导向的工作和完成任务的经验非常有限，而且该员工需要有监督、委托、在职的增量任务，并定期进行指导和反馈
2	新手从业者	已任职1年或1年以上，正在发展相关职责领域的能力，但除最基本的委派专业任务外，其他所有任务仍需在督导和监督下完成
3	独立从业者	在特定领域具有独立和可靠的能力。只有在少数特殊或例外情况下，才需要寻求建议或指导
4	高级从业者	已掌握该领域的知识。是公认的专家，并通过研究、实验和创新拓展领域知识的边界。被公认为后辈的培训师和导师，被同行和其他人寻求技术建议和指导

■ Annex 3

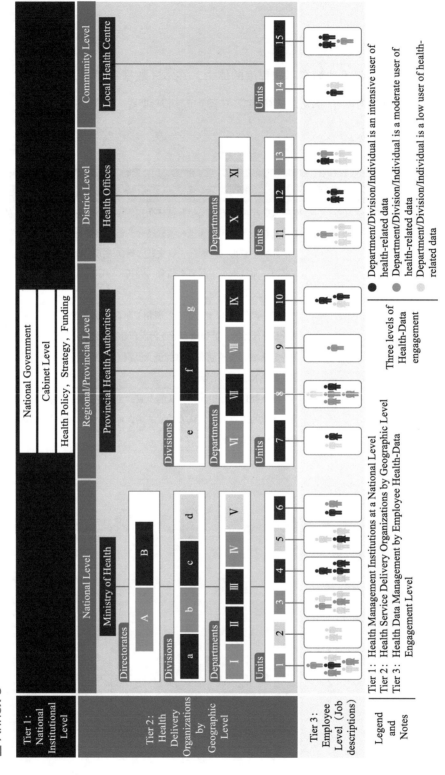

Tier 1: Health Management Institutions at a National Level
Tier 2: Health Service Delivery Organizations by Geographic Level
Tier 3: Health Data Management by Employee Health-Data Engagement Level

● Department/Division/Individual is an intensive user of health-related data
● Department/Division/Individual is a moderate user of health-related data
○ Department/Division/Individual is a low user of health-related data

Three levels of Health-Data engagement

■ 附件 3

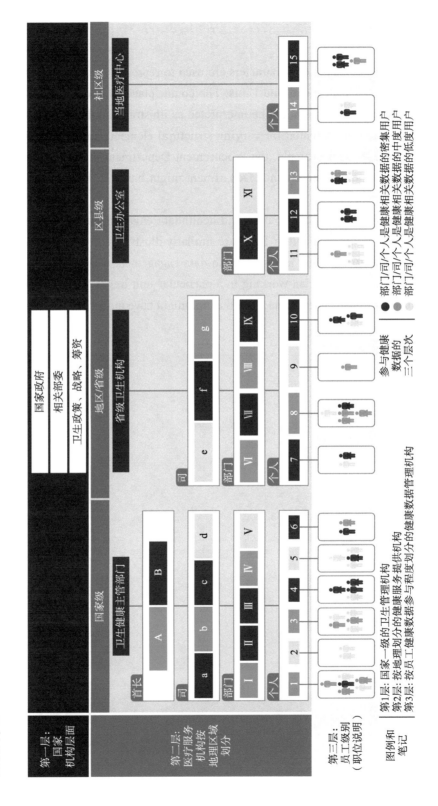

第一层：
国家/
机构层面

| 国家政府 |
| 相关部委 |
| 卫生政策、战略、筹资 |

第二层：
医疗服务
机构按
地理区域
划分

第三层：
员工级别
（职位说明）

图例和
笔记

第1层：国家一级的卫生管理机构
第2层：按地理划分的医疗服务提供机构
第3层：按员工健康数据参与程度划分的健康数据管理机构

● 部门与个人是健康相关数据的密集用户
● 部门与个人是健康相关数据的中度用户
● 部门与个人是健康相关数据的低度用户

参与健康
数据的
三个层次

National Health Sector Architecture Mapping, by Health-Data Engagement

The alphanumeric characters are used to represent "real world" Directorates/Divisions/Departments and Units. The count, placement and healthdata engagement classifications should be interpreted as illustrative rather than prescriptive, indicating the potential for varying structural elements and health-data engagement levels (for example, the Procurement Department might have low engagement while the Surveillance Department might have intensive engagement with health data).

The number, distribution and healthdata engagement classification of employees under each unit in Tier 3 are similarly illustrative in use to demonstrate the potential for different levels of health-data engagement within a common unit (for example, a statistician working in a particular unit might have intensive engagement, while the team manager of the unit might have moderate engagement).

按卫生数据参与情况绘制国家卫生部门架构图

· 字母数字字符用于代表"现实世界"中的首长、司、部门和个人。计数、位置和健康数据参与度分类应被理解为说明性而非规范性的，表明可能存在不同的结构要素和健康数据参与度水平（例如，采购部的参与度可能较低，而监督部可能对健康数据的参与度较高）

· 第3层中各单位下员工的数量、分布和健康数据参与度分类同样具有说明性，可用于表明共同单位内不同健康数据参与度的可能性（例如，在特定单位工作的统计员可能具有密集参与度，而该单位的团队经理可能具有中等参与度）。

References

1. Fagherazzi G, Goetzinger C, Rashid M, Aguayo G, Huiart L. Digital health strategies to fight COVID-19 worldwide: Challenges, recommendations, and a call for papers. J Med Internet Res. 2020; 22 (6): e19284. doi: 10.2196/19284

2. Implementing telemedicine services during COVID-19: guiding principles and considerations for a stepwise approach. Manila: WHO Regional Office for the Western Pacific; 2020 (https: //apps.who.int/iris/handle/10665/336862, accessed 27 October 2022).

3. Whitepaper 2022: Examining today's HIM workforce with recommendations for elevating the profession. IFHIMA; 2022 (https: //ifhimasitemedia.s3.us-east-2.amazonaws.com/wp-content/uploads/2022/10/24142247/IFHIMA_Workforce_WP_2022_FINAL.pdf, accessed 25 October 2022).

4. Michener WK. Ten simple rules for creating a good data management plan. PLoS Comput Biol. 2015; 11 (10): e1004525. doi: https: //doi.org/10.1371/journal.pcbi.1004525

5. Data management guide: Crafting your data management plan. In: Research data [website]. Cambridge: University of Cambridge; 2022 (https: //www.data.cam.ac.uk/data-management-guide/creating-your-data/data-management-plan, accessed 26 October 2022).

6. Burnette MH, Williams SC, Imker HJ. From plan to action: Successful data management plan implementation in a multidisciplinary project. J Escience Librariansh. 2016; 5 (1): e1101. doi: 10.7191/jeslib.2016.1101

7. Bartlett R. A practitioner's guide to business analytics: Using data analysis tools to improve your organization's decision making and strategy. New York (NY): McGraw Hill Professional; 2013.

8. Pasquale E, Canton A. Clinical audit, a valuable tool to improve quality of care: General methodology and applications in nephrology. World Journal of Nephrology. 2014 Nov 6; 3 (4): 249-55. doi: 10.5527/wjn.v3.i4.249. PMID: 25374819; PMCID: PMC4220358.

9. Watson RT. Data management: Databases and organizations, sixth edition. Burlington (VT): Prospect Press; 2016.

10. Plotkin D. Data stewardship. An actionable guide to effective data management and data governance. Amsterdam: Elsevier/Morgan Kaufman; 2014.

11. Provost F, Fawcett T. Data science for business. Sebastopol (CA): O'Reilly Media Inc.; 2013.

12. Briney K. Data management for researchers: Organize, maintain, and share your data for research success. Exeter: Pelagic Publishing; 2015.

13. Maheshwari A. Data analytics made accessible. North Charleston (SC): CreateSpace Independent Publishing Platform; 2014.

14. Zio MD, Fursova NY, Gelsema T, Giessing S, Guarnera U, Petrauskienė J, et al. Methodology for data validation 1.0. Brussels: European Commission, The ESSnet ValiDat Foundation; 2016. (https: //ec.europa.eu/eurostat/cros/system/files/methodology_for_data_validation_v1.0_rev-2016-06_final.pdf).

—— **参 考 文 献** ——

15. Harvard Business School Publishing Corporation. HBR guide to data analytics for managers. Boston（MA）：Harvard Business Review Press; 2018.

16. Baha H. An introduction to descriptive analysis; Its advantages and disadvantages ［online assignment］. 2017.（https：//www.academia.edu/25307454/, accessed 25 October 2022）.

17. Robertson T. What is diagnostic analysis［website］. The Data Science Academy; 2020 https：//www.datascienceacademy.io/blog/what-is-diagnostic-analysis; -steps-to-do-this/, accessed 25 October）.

18. Sarmento R, Costa V. Descriptive analysis. In：Sarmento R, Costa V, editors. Comparative approaches to using R and Python for statistical data analysis. Hershey （PA）：IGI Global; 2017. DOI：10.4018/978-1-68318-016-6.ch004.（https：//www.researchgate.net/publication/345213754_Descriptive_Analysis/, accessed 25 October 2022）

19. Theobald O. Data analytics for absolute beginners：A deconstructed guide to data literacy, second edition. Independently published; 2019.

20. Dursun D. Prescriptive analytics：The final frontier for evidence-based management and optimal decision making, first edition. Hoboken（NJ）：Pearson Education Inc; 2020.

21. Trochim WMK. The research methods knowledge base：Inferential statistics［web-based textbook］. Hosted by conjointly.com; version current as of 25 October 2022 （https：//conjointly.com/kb/inferential-statistics/）.

22. Gates M. Machine learning：Step-by-step guide simplified. North Charleston（SC）：CreateSpace Independent Publishing Platform; 2017.

23. Hutcheson GD, Moutinho L. Statistical modelling for management. London：SAGE Publications Ltd; 2008.

24. Mendis A. Statistical modelling vs machine learning［website］. KDnuggets; 2019 （https：//www.kdnuggets.com/2019/08/statistical-modelling-vs-machine-learning. html, accessed 25 October 2022）.

25. Schünemann HJ, Vist GE, Higgins JPT, Santesso N, Deeks JJ, Glasziou P, et al. Chapter 15：Interpreting results and drawing conclusions. In：Higgins JPT, Thomas J, Chandler J, Cumpston M, Li T, Page M, Welch VA, editors. Cochrane handbook for systematic reviews of interventions. London：Cochrane; February 2022（www. training.cochrane.org/handbook）.

26. Adapted and contextualised from Merriam-Webster［online dictionary］; version current as of 25 October 2022.（https：//www.merriam-webster.com）.

27. Crago J. Interpreting data and understanding your findings［website］. Published online on Mackman Research; version current as of 25 October 2022.（https：//www. mackmanresearch.co.uk/interpreting-data-and-findings/）.

28. Field B, Booth A, Ilott I, Gerrish K. Using the Knowledge to Action Framework in practice：A citation analysis and systematic review. Implementation Science. 2014; 9 （172）. DOI：https：//doi.org/10.1186/s13012-014-0172-2.